Orofacial Trauma and Emergency Care

Guest Editors

SAMI M.A. CHOGLE, BDS, DMD, MSD
GERALD A. FERRETTI, DDS, MS, MPH

DENTAL CLINICS OF NORTH AMERICA

www.dental.theclinics.com

October 2009 • Volume 53 • Number 4

SAUNDERS an imprint of ELSEVIER, Inc.

W.B. SAUNDERS COMPANY
A Division of Elsevier Inc.

1600 John F. Kennedy Boulevard ● Suite 1800 ● Philadelphia, Pennsylvania 19103-2899

http://www.dental.theclinics.com

DENTAL CLINICS OF NORTH AMERICA Volume 53, Number 4
October 2009 ISSN 0011-8532, ISBN-13: 978-1-4377-1208-7, ISBN-10: 1-4377-1208-8

Editor: John Vassallo; j.vassallo@elsevier.com
Developmental Editor: Theresa Collier

Dental Clinics of North America (ISSN 0011-8532) is published quarterly by Elsevier Inc., 360 Park Avenue South, New York, NY 10010-1710. Months of issue are January, April, July, and October. Business and Editorial Offices: 1600 John F. Kennedy Boulevard, Suite 1800, Philadelphia, PA 19103-2899. Periodicals postage paid at New York, NY and additional mailing offices. Subscription prices are $224.00 per year (domestic individuals), $382.00 per year (domestic institutions), $108.00 per year (domestic students/residents), $266.00 per year (Canadian individuals), $481.00 per year (Canadian institutions), $321.00 per year (international individuals), $481.00 per year (international institutions), and $162.00 per year (international and Canadian students/residents. International air speed delivery is included in all *Clinics* subscription prices. All prices are subject to change without notice. **POSTMASTER:** Send address changes to *Dental Clinics of North America*, Elsevier Health Sciences Division, Subscription Customer Service, 3251 Riverport Lane, Maryland Heights, MO 63043. **Customer Service (orders, claims, online, change of address): Elsevier Health Sciences Division, Subscription Customer Service, 3251 Riverport Lane, Maryland Heights, MO 63043. Tel: 1-800-654-2452 (U.S. and Canada). Fax: 314-447-8029. E-mail: journalscustomerservice-usa@elsevier.com (for print support); journalsonlinesupport-usa@elsevier.com (for online support).**

Reprints. For copies of 100 or more, of articles in this publication, please contact the Commercial Reprints Department, Elsevier Inc., 360 Park Avenue South, New York, NY 10010-1710. Tel.: 212-633-3812; Fax: 212-462-1935; E-mail: reprints@elsevier.com.

The *Dental Clinics of North America* is covered in *MEDLINE/PubMed (Index Medicus), Current Contents/Clinical Medicine, ISI/BIOMED* and *Clinahl.*

Printed and bound by CPI Group (UK) Ltd, Croydon, CR0 4YY

Transferred to Digital Print 2011

Contributors

GUEST EDITORS

SAMI M.A. CHOGLE, BDS, DMD, MSD
Associate Professor, Department of Endodontics, School of Dental Medicine, Case Western Reserve University, Cleveland, Ohio; Associate Professor, Department of Endodontics, Henry M. Goldman School of Dental Medicine, Boston University, Boston, Massachusetts; Associate Professor and Program Director, Department of Endodontics, Institute of Dental Research and Education, Boston University, Dubai, United Arab Emirates

GERALD A. FERRETTI, DDS, MS, MPH
Professor, Pediatric Dentistry and Pediatrics; Chief of Dentistry, Rainbow Babies and Children's Hospital, Cleveland, Ohio; Chair of Pediatric Dentistry, School of Dental Medicine, Case Western Reserve University, Cleveland, Ohio

AUTHORS

A. OMAR ABUBAKER, DMD, PhD
Professor and Chairman, Department of Oral and Maxillofacial Surgery, Virginia Commonwealth University School of Dentistry and Virginia Commonwealth University Medical Center, Richmond, Virginia

LEIF K. BAKLAND, DDS
Professor, Department of Endodontics, School of Dentistry, Loma Linda University, Loma Linda, California

DALE A. BAUR, DDS, MD
Associate Professor and Chair, Department of Oral and Maxillofacial Surgery, Case Western Reserve University, Cleveland, Ohio

CECILIA BOURGUIGNON, DDS
Endodontics and Dental Traumatology Clinic, Paris, France

SAMI M.A. CHOGLE, BDS, DMD, MSD
Associate Professor, Department of Endodontics, School of Dental Medicine, Case Western Reserve University, Cleveland, Ohio; Associate Professor, Department of Endodontics, Henry M. Goldman School of Dental Medicine, Boston University, Boston, Massachusetts; Associate Professor and Program Director, Department of Endodontics, Institute of Dental Research and Education, Boston University, Dubai, United Arab Emirates

HUSAM ELIAS, MD, DMD
Staff Oral and Maxillofacial Surgeon, Head and Neck Institute, Cleveland Clinic, Cleveland, Ohio

DAVID E. JARAMILLO, DDS
Assistant Professor and Clinic Director of Endodontics, School of Dentistry, Loma Linda University, Loma Linda, California

DENNIS J. McTIGUE, DDS, MS
Professor, Division of Pediatric Dentistry, The Ohio State University College of Dentistry, Columbus, Ohio

ALEX J. MOULE, BDSc, PhD
Endodontist and Associate Professor, University of Queensland, Brisbane, Queensland, Australia

CHRISTOPHER A. MOULE, BDSc
General Practitioner, Queensland, Australia

LEENA PALOMO, DDS, MSD
Diplomate, American Board of Periodontology; Assistant Professor and Director of Undergraduate Periodontics, Department of Periodontics, Case School of Dental Medicine, Case Western Reserve University, Cleveland, Ohio

J. MARTIN PALOMO, DDS, MSD
Diplomate, American Board of Orthodontics; Associate Professor and Program Director in the Department of Orthodontics, Case School of Dental Medicine, Cleveland, Ohio; Director of Craniofacial Imaging Center, Case School of Dental Medicine, Case Western Reserve University, Cleveland, Ohio

ASGEIR SIGURDSSON, DDS, MS
Private Practice, Reykjavik, Iceland

PANAGIOTIS K. STEFANOPOULOS, DDS, LT COL (DC)
Hellenic Army, Oral and Maxillofacial Surgery Department, Athens, Greece

KUMAR SUBRAMANIAN, DDS, MSD
Private Practice and Department of Dentistry, Nationwide Children's Hospital, Columbus, Ohio

ANDROMACHE D. TARANTZOPOULOU, DDS
Department of Periodontology and Implant Biology, Dental School, Aristotle University of Thessaloniki, Thessaloniki, Greece

Contents

Medical and Orofacial Considerations in Traumatic Dental Injuries

Kumar Subramanian and Sami M.A. Chogle

A complete medical and dental evaluation is imperative following traumatic dental injuries, which are emergent situations that need a quick assessment and appropriate management. The proper diagnosis and treatment rendered determines the prognosis of the case. Proper documentation is important for medicolegal reasons and for baseline reference regarding the traumatic injury. Future treatment modalities and outcomes can be better managed with accurate documentation at the initial assessment.

Managing Injuries to the Primary Dentition

Dennis J. McTigue

This article overviews the diagnosis and management of traumatic injuries to primary teeth. The child's age, ability to cooperate for treatment, and the potential for collateral damage to developing permanent teeth can complicate the management of these injuries. The etiology of these injuries is reviewed including the disturbing role of child abuse. Serious medical complications including head injury, cervical spine injury, and tetanus are discussed. Diagnostic methods and the rationale for treatment of luxation injuries, crown, and crown/root fractures are included. Treatment priorities should include adequate pain control, safe management of the child's behavior, and protection of the developing permanent teeth.

Minor Traumatic Injuries to the Permanent Dentition

Alex J. Moule and Christopher A. Moule

Treatment of traumatized teeth generally occurs in two phases: short-term emergency treatment and stabilization followed by endodontic management and review. These authors recently reviewed the endodontic considerations in the treatment of traumatized permanent anterior teeth, and in this article review the early management of traumatized permanent teeth. Preoperative assessment and emergency management are emphasized, as is the treatment of immature teeth for which continued development of the root system must be encouraged. Factors influencing long-term prognosis are discussed and the influence of various management strategies evaluated.

Revisiting Traumatic Pulpal Exposure: Materials, Management Principles, and Techniques

Leif K. Bakland

This article presents current concepts of managing teeth with traumatic pulp exposures. The article includes a description of the traumatology of

crown fractures, discussion of treatment considerations, a summary of
materials for vital pulp therapy, and an outline of techniques for treating
pulp exposures.

Teeth, periodontium, and supporting alveolar bone are frequently involved
in trauma and account for approximately 15% of all emergency room
visits. The cause of the dentoalveolar trauma varies in different demographics but generally results from falls, playground accidents, domestic
violence, bicycle accidents, motor vehicle accidents, assaults, altercations, and sports injuries. Dentoalveolar injuries should be considered an
emergency situation because successful management of the injury
requires proper diagnosis and treatment within a limited time to achieve
better outcomes.

Bite wounds are especially prone to infectious complications, both local
and systemic. In bite wounds to the face, such complications can create
more difficulties than the initial tissue damage itself for the task of restoring
an esthetic appearance. Management should aim to neutralize this potential for infection and provide an infection-free environment for wound healing. Wound cleansing followed by primary closure is the treatment of
choice, and the use of prophylactic antibiotics may further decrease the
risk of infection. Delay in presentation beyond 24 hours is not necessarily
a contraindication to immediate repair, but excessive crushing of the tissues or extensive edema usually dictates a more conservative approach,
such as delayed closure.

In managing traumatic wounds, the primary goal is to achieve rapid healing
with optimal functional and esthetic results. This is best accomplished by
providing an environment that prevents infection of the wound during healing. Despite good wound care, some infections still occur. Accordingly,
some investigators argue that prophylactic antibiotics have an important
role in the management of certain types of wounds. This article reviews
the basis of antibiotic use in preventing wound infection in general and
its use in oral and facial wounds in particular.

Three-dimensional imaging offers many advantages in making diagnoses
and planning treatment. This article focuses on cone beam CT (CBCT) for

making diagnoses and planning treatment in trauma-related cases. CBCT equipment is smaller and less expensive than traditional medical CT equipment and is tailored to address challenges specific to the dentoalveolar environment. Like medical CT, CBCT offers a three-dimensional view that conventional two-dimensional dental radiography fails to provide. CBCT combines the strengths of medical CT with those of conventional dental radiography to accommodate unique diagnostic and treatment-planning applications that have particular utility in dentoalveolar trauma cases. CBCT is useful, for example, in identifying tooth fractures relative to surrounding alveolar bone, in determining alveolar fracture location and morphology, in analyzing ridge-defect height and width, and in imaging temporomandibular joints. Treatment-planning applications include those involving extraction of fractured teeth, placement of implants, exposure of impacted teeth, and analyses of airways.

Traumatic dental and maxillofacial injuries are common occurrences, and affect worldwide approximately 20% to 30% of permanent dentition, often with serious aesthetic, functional, psychological, and economic consequences. With such a high frequency of injuries, prevention becomes a primary goal. A prevention approach relies on the identification of etiologic factors, and on giving rise to measures aimed at avoiding those factors or at reducing their impact. This article reviews the etiology and preventive strategy regarding dental injuries, and examines the role and manufacture of appliances, especially mouthguards, in preventive dentistry.

The old Boy Scout's motto, "Be Prepared," can be beneficially applied to the management of dental trauma. A large number of dental injuries occur every year, primarily in the 7- to 15-year age group. Preserving the natural dentition during that time period is critically important, because tooth loss at an early age presents significant lifelong dental problems. Being prepared to manage an emergency can make the difference between tooth loss and a successful outcome. Two factors contribute to achieving the better outcome: knowledge of the essentials of dental traumatology, and being prepared with the dental materials needed for appropriate treatment. It is the hope of the authors that these factors are clearly elucidated in this article.

RELATED INTEREST

Oral and Maxillofacial Surgery Clinics of North America May 2009 (Vol. 21, No. 2)
Current Controversies in Maxillofacial Trauma
Daniel M. Laskin, DDS, MS, and A. Omar Abubaker, DMD, PhD, *Guest Editors*

THE CLINICS ARE NOW AVAILABLE ONLINE!

Access your subscription at:
www.theclinics.com

Preface

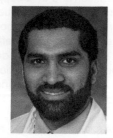
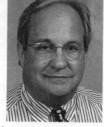

Sami M.A. Chogle, BDS, DMD, MSD   Gerald A. Ferretti, DDS, MS, MPH
Guest Editors

In this issue of *Dental Clinics of North America* devoted to orofacial trauma and emergency care, we present current understanding of the nature of dental trauma, preventive strategies, and subsequent healing and treatment modalities.

As Drs J.O. Andreasen, F.M. Andreasen, and L. Andersson prefaced in their *Textbook and Color Atlas of Traumatic Injuries to the Teeth,* "The study and understanding of healing in hard and soft tissues after trauma is probably one of the most serious challenges facing the dental profession. That this task presently rests with only a handful of researchers is out of proportion with the fact that perhaps half of the world's population today has suffered oral or dental trauma." Furthermore, such patients presenting with acute dental trauma report to the dental clinic unexpectedly. As dental clinicians, we need to be prepared and current on dental trauma and its emergent care.

Thanks to brilliant inquisitive minds and their published research, we have come a long way since the early 1970s in understanding dental trauma and defining treatment strategies. Several events first deemed as requiring aggressive treatment have not been supported by thorough current research. All the contributors to this issue share a commitment to the principles and practice of evidence-based health care. They approach this subject from a variety of viewpoints. There are examples of best practices based on a high level of evidence, and there are also examples of how to proceed when high-quality evidence is lacking. Due to the fact that the treatment approach in itself is usually traumatogenic, treatment principles for traumatized teeth become critical. In the case of some trauma entities, such as concussion, subluxation, and some injuries to the primary dentition, observation and follow-up is the only treatment needed. In other situations, repositioning and splinting procedures characterize treatment. Techniques for the reduction of tooth dislocations include immediate digital repositioning and orthodontic or surgical repositioning. Recent research suggests that the selection of treatment modality should be very specific and related to preinjury or injury factors to optimize healing.

The purpose of this issue is to provide the clinician, whether in a dental practice or emergency service of a hospital, with an understanding of acute dental trauma,

Dent Clin N Am 53 (2009) ix–xi
doi:10.1016/j.cden.2009.08.002
0011-8532/09/$ – see front matter © 2009 Elsevier Inc. All rights reserved.

preventive strategies, and current treatment approaches. In that regard, the articles in this issue follow a sequence of medical and physical evaluation, classification and biology of traumatic injuries to the primary and permanent dentition and their supporting structures, preventive strategies, and acute and long-term treatment modalities. In most cases, a traumatic event involves more than the dentition and its supporting structures. Therefore, the dental clinician must be able to evaluate systemic effects of the injury. In the past decade, better understanding of the biology of the dental pulp and the use of new materials and techniques have opened new possibilities for management of pulpal exposures. Injuries to the alveolus, maxilla, and/or mandible complicate healing and need longer and more customized treatment plans. These topics are fully covered in articles in this issue.

Acute dental trauma implies severe pain and psychological impact for many patients. The choice of treatment may be different for injuries to primary and permanent dentition depending on several factors, including type of injury, age, and tooth type. In the likely event that most dentists will end up treating traumatic injuries on an emergency basis, the astute clinician will develop a dental trauma kit for such situations. The dental clinicians must also provide information as to the prevention of dental injuries, including accident-prone sports activities where mouth guards could be of value. Several articles in this issue deal with these subjects.

In the wake of esthetically and functionally successful implant therapy, information has been included on implants as part of oral rehabilitation, with a discussion of the primary biologic principles and the use of implants after dental trauma. This is important as a much longer treatment solution because these patients are often young children in whom the placement of an implant is contraindicated because it interferes with growth and development of the jaw.

We thank the authors for their time and effort in making this issue of the *Dental Clinics of North America* a current and comprehensive aid to the dental clinician and providing the rationale and methods of optimal care to the acutely traumatized patient. It is also hoped that these articles will provide the stimulus for further reading in the field. Those interested in an in-depth discussion of the epidemiology, psychological and biological impact of the various trauma entities on the pulp and periodontium, the pathogenesis of the various healing complications, and long-term effects and treatment of oral trauma are referred to the *Textbook and Color Atlas of Traumatic Injuries to the Teeth*, 4th edition.

Sami M.A. Chogle, BDS, DMD, MSD
Department of Endodontics
School of Dental Medicine
Case Western Reserve University
10900 Euclid Avenue
Cleveland, OH 44106, USA

Department of Endodontics
Henry M. Golden School of Dental Medicine
Boston University
100 East Newton Street G-305
Boston, MA 02118, USA

Department of Endodontics
Institute for Dental Research and Education
Boston University
Dubai Health-Care City
Building #34, Al-Zahrawi Complex
PO Box 505097, Dubai, UAE

Gerald A. Ferretti, DDS, MS, MPH
Rainbow Babies and Children's Hospital
Cleveland, OH, USA

School of Dental Medicine
Case Western Reserve University
10900 Euclid Avenue
Cleveland, OH, USA

E-mail addresses:
sxc89@case.edu (S.M.A. Chogle)
gaf10@case.edu (G.A. Ferretti)

Medical and Orofacial Considerations in Traumatic Dental Injuries

Kumar Subramanian, DDS, MSD[a],*, Sami M.A. Chogle, BDS, DDS, MSD[b]

KEYWORDS

- Emergency • Cranio-facial • Laceration • Bleeding • Vitality

A complete medical and dental evaluation is imperative following traumatic dental injuries. Traumatic dental injuries are emergent situations that need a quick assessment and appropriate management. The proper diagnosis and treatment rendered determines the prognosis of the case. It is also important to have proper documentation, not only for medicolegal reasons but to have a baseline reference regarding the traumatic injury. Future treatment modalities and outcomes can be better managed with accurate documentation at the initial assessment.

MEDICAL CONSIDERATIONS

A comprehensive medical evaluation of the patient with traumatic dental injuries is required before any dental treatment is rendered. Patients with trauma may present with extensive injuries, some of which may be life-threatening, or they may have some preexisting medical condition that may affect the overall dental treatment.[1] A complete medical evaluation is usually performed by the physician. However, the treating dental clinician should be in a position to evaluate the general medical issues that may affect the emergency dental care to be provided.

A detailed medical history should be taken as soon as possible. The clinician should review all systemic diseases, medications taken, allergies, hospitalizations, and other relevant points. Vital signs should be recorded. As the trauma is to the orofacial region, a quick evaluation of the respiratory and circulatory system should be done to confirm normal breathing and circulation.

[a] Department of Dentistry, Nationwide Children's Hospital, Columbus, Ohio, USA
[b] Department of Endodontics, Case Western Reserve University, 10900 Euclid Avenue, Cleveland, OH 44106-4905, USA
* Corresponding author.
E-mail address: ksubr2@email.uky.edu (K. Subramanian).

Dent Clin N Am 53 (2009) 617–626
doi:10.1016/j.cden.2009.08.001
0011-8532/09/$ – see front matter © 2009 Published by Elsevier Inc.

dental.theclinics.com

Shock, an important complication that is often associated with traumatic injuries, is indicated by pale skin, cool extremities, excess perspiration, tachycardia, hypotension, and confused state. The most common type is hypovolemic shock due to hemorrhage. Facial fractures, however, rarely cause life-threatening hemorrhage. The presence of physical injuries and facial asymmetry should be recorded.

Traumatic injuries may also result in a partial or complete airway obstruction due to the aspiration of avulsed teeth, tooth fragments, or removable prosthesis.[2] The common signs and symptoms include coughing, cyanosis, and dyspnea. Any suspicion of aspiration or airway obstruction should be evaluated with a radiograph of the chest, to rule out a foreign body in the lungs. A radiograph of the abdomen is also indicated in patients with missing teeth or prosthesis.

The patient's clinical status at the time of presentation following a traumatic incident should be assessed using the Glasgow Coma Scale (**Table 1**),[3] which helps the clinician determine the presence of any brain injury. The scale assigns numerical values for eye openings and various motor and verbal responses that indicate the level of consciousness and extent of dysfunction. The scores range from 3 to 15 and lower scores indicate more extensive brain injury. Bradycardia with hypertension may indicate increased intracranial pressure. A history of loss of consciousness, dizziness, headache, nausea, and vomiting could also indicate possible intracranial injury, necessitating immediate medical attention.

A cursory neurologic examination of the patient should be performed to assess any potential life threatening issues that need emergency medical care. A failure to recognize an emergency situation may lead to a rapid deterioration of the patient's condition. Breathing difficulty, hypotension, raised intracranial pressure, disorientation, loss of consciousness, seizures, severe headache, nausea, or vomiting and amnesia are all possible signs of intracranial injury, which requires immediate hospitalization for emergency medical care.

Another serious situation necessitating immediate care is craniofacial fracture, leading to leakage of cerebrospinal fluid through the nose (rhinorrhea) or the ear (otorrhea).[4] This may be due to the fracture of the anterior cranial base or the posterior wall of the frontal sinus.

A thorough examination of all the cranial nerves should be done to rule out any underlying injury. Diplopia is often a complication of fracture of the zygomaticomaxillary complex. The ability of the patient to open and close eyes and the pupillary reaction to light help determine underlying neurologic injury. If cervical vertebral injury exists, the patient should be immobilized and referred for immediate medical care. Protrusion and any deflection of the tongue suggest possible damage to the hypoglossal nerve. The ability of the patient to maintain postural balance and hear normally helps assess the vestibulocochlear nerve. The presence or absence of paresthesia or anesthesia on localized areas of the face helps determine any damage to the trigeminal nerve with associated facial fractures (**Table 2**).

SOFT TISSUE EXAMINATION

A thorough examination of the extraoral and intraoral soft tissue should be done during the initial visit. The presence and location of lacerations, contusions, or tissue abrasions should be noted and the areas gently washed and cleaned with antiseptics. Bleeding and larger wounds may necessitate suturing. Any asymmetry or distinct change in the facial appearance should be noted and followed up by clinical and radiographic examination for possible fractures.

Table 1
Glasgow Coma Scale assessment

	1	2	3	4	5	6
Eyes	Does not open eyes	Opens eyes in response to painful stimuli	Opens eyes in response to voice	Opens eyes spontaneously	NA	NA
Verbal	Makes no sounds	Incomprehensible sounds	Utters inappropriate words	Confused, disorientated	Oriented, converses normally	NA
Motor	Makes no movements	Extension to painful stimuli	Abnormal flexion to painful stimuli	Flexion/withdrawal to painful stimuli	Localizes painful stimuli	Obeys commands

Abbreviation: NA, not applicable.

Table 2
Cranial nerves evaluation

Cranial Nerve Number	Name	Function	Test
1	Olfactory	Smell	The ability to smell is tested by asking the person to identify items with specific odors (such as soap, coffee, and cloves) that are placed under the nose. Each nostril is tested separately
2	Optic	Vision and detection of light	The ability to see is tested by asking the person to read an eye chart. Peripheral vision is tested by asking the person to detect objects or movement from the corners of the eyes. The ability to detect light is tested by shining a bright light (as from a flashlight) into each pupil in a darkened room.
3	Oculomotor	Eye movement upward, downward, and inward Narrowing (constriction) or widening (dilation) of the pupil in response to changes in light Raises the eyelids	The ability to move each eye up, down, and inward is tested by asking the person to follow a target moved by the examiner The pupils' response to light is checked by shining a bright light (as from a flashlight) into each pupil in a darkened room The upper eyelid is checked for drooping (ptosis)
4	Trochlear	Eye movement downward and inward	The ability to move each eye down and inward is tested by asking the person to follow a target moved by the examiner
5	Trigeminal	Facial sensation and chewing	Sensation in areas of the face is tested using a pin and a wisp of cotton. The blink reflex is tested by touching the cornea of the eye with a cotton wisp. Strength and movement of muscles that control the jaw are tested by asking the person to clench the teeth and open the jaw against resistance

#	Nerve	Function	Test
6	Abducens	Eye movement outward	The ability to move each eye outward beyond the midline is tested by asking the person to look to the side
7	Facial	Facial expression, taste in the front two-thirds of the tongue, and production of saliva and tears	The ability to move the face is tested by asking the person to smile, to open the mouth and show the teeth, and to close the eyes tightly. Taste is tested using substances that are sweet (sugar), sour (lemon juice), salty (salt), and bitter (aspirin, quinine, or aloes)
8	Auditory (vestibulocochlear)	Hearing and balance	Hearing is tested with a tuning fork or with headphones that play tones of different frequencies (pitches) and loudness (audiometry). Balance is tested by asking the person to walk in a straight line
9	Glossopharyngeal	Swallowing, gag reflex, and speech	Because the 9th and 10th cranial nerves control similar functions, they are tested together. The person is asked to swallow; to say "ah-h-h", to check movement of the palate (roof of the mouth) and uvula (small, soft projection that hangs down at the back of throat). The back of the throat may be touched with a tongue blade, which evokes the gag reflex in most people. The person is asked to speak to determine whether the voice sounds nasal
10	Vagus	Swallowing, gag reflex, and speech / Control of muscle in internal organs (including the heart)	
11	Accessory	Neck turning and shoulder shrugging	The person is asked to turn the head and to shrug the shoulders against resistance provided by the examiner
12	Hypoglossal	Tongue movement	The person is asked to stick out the tongue, which is observed for deviation to one side or the other

INTRAORAL EXAMINATION

Examination of intraoral tissue should be done in an orderly manner to avoid missing any detail. Intraoral tissue is highly vascular and even minor injuries may cause significant bleeding that could preclude a proper examination of the underlying tissue. Careful rinsing and suction of the oral cavity should precede evaluation of the tissue. Lacerations and penetrating injuries[5] should be carefully explored for possible tooth fragments or other debris[6] that is lodged within the tissue (**Fig. 1**). The presence of a swelling on palpation of the soft tissue may indicate embedded tooth fragments or debris.

When there is excessive bleeding from the soft tissue, firm pressure should be applied with sterile gauze to arrest the bleeding. If this is not sufficient, then tissue should be anesthetized using a local anesthetic with a vasoconstrictor and sutured carefully. Once the bleeding is controlled, further examination of oral tissue should be done (**Fig. 2**).

The soft tissue of the periodontium should also be carefully scrutinized for evidence of bleeding from the sulcus. This may indicate a tooth displacement, a crown-root fracture, or an alveolar fracture. The maxilla and the mandible should be examined for the presence of fractures (**Fig. 3**).

RADIOGRAPHIC EXAMINATION

The presence of hematoma, facial asymmetry, deviation of the mandible, or swelling or crepitus on palpation is suggestive of probable fracture and necessitates radiographic evaluation of the affected areas. Pain, malocclusion, and mobility of the fracture's segments are further evidence of fractures. However, in the event of favorable fractures, there may be no evidence of malocclusion or mobility of the fracture's segments. Hence, radiographs should be carefully inspected. The advent of cone beam technology helps the definitive diagnosis of these conditions.

The presence of embedded tooth fragments or debris in the soft tissue should also be evaluated with radiographs. In the case of soft-tissue radiographic examination, a lowered dose, with appropriate film or sensor placement, may be necessary.

TEETH
Examination

Trauma to the orofacial region always necessitates a thorough clinical examination of the teeth. Adverse events include missing, displaced, fractured, or avulsed teeth. Depending on the extent of displacement, treatment may be warranted immediately or at

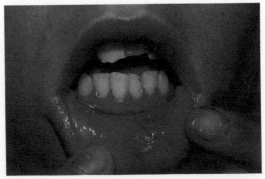

Fig. 1. Tooth fragment in lip. (*Courtesy of* Dennis J. McTigue, DDS, MS, Columbus, OH, USA.)

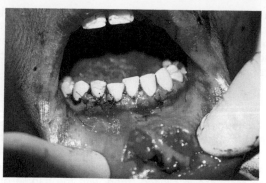

Fig. 2. Lip laceration. (*Courtesy of* Dennis J. McTigue, DDS, MS, Columbus, OH, USA.)

a later date, as recommended by the International Association of Dental Traumatology (IADT) guidelines.[7]

The extent of damage to the tooth or teeth should be assessed clinically. A radiographic examination should follow to identify the presence and extent of displacement of the tooth and to verify the stage of root development. This will aid in the treatment plan of the traumatized tooth.

The presence of cracks or minor Class I and II fractures may result in hypersensitivity. The careful clinical examination of the affected teeth and adjacent ones should be done with proper illumination and magnification. The affected teeth should also be examined by transillumination. Any asymmetry should be noted and, if needed, the affected tooth or teeth repositioned. When fractures exist, patients should be evaluated for pulp exposure; if present, the size and location of pulp exposure should be documented. A palliative approach to alleviating discomfort in the absence of pulp exposure, without traumatizing the tooth further, would be the application of an adhesive bandage (Band-Aid). In the event of pulpal involvement, appropriate treatment should be followed, as provided in the IADT guidelines.

Mobility

The mobility of the tooth is carefully checked by moving the tooth between 2 instruments (mouth mirror handles), and the degree of mobility is documented.

0—no mobility
+1—less than or equal to 1 mm of horizontal movement
+2—more than 1 mm of horizontal movement
+3—more than 1 mm of horizontal movement and depressible in the socket

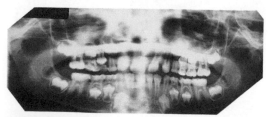

Fig. 3. Bilateral condylar fracture. (*Courtesy of* Dennis J. McTigue, DDS, MS, Columbus, OH, USA.)

Teeth that have undergone subluxation, luxation, or extrusion injuries tend to exhibit increased mobility, whereas teeth that are intruded may show a complete lack of mobility. The presence of moderate-to-severe mobility necessitates splinting of the affected teeth to adjacent teeth for stabilization and for prevention of further damage to the attachment apparatus.

Percussion

The percussion test determines the presence or absence of periradicular periodontitis. Inflammation around the apical fibers of the periodontal ligament surrounding the root surface will result in varying degrees of discomfort on percussion of the affected tooth. To minimize discomfort, percussion should be done by gentle tapping, initially with the fingertips, and if no response is elicited, then with the handle of a mouth mirror. Percussion should be done in a vertical and lateral direction to diagnose damage to the periodontal ligament. If a tooth is intruded or ankylosed, percussion will produce a dull metallic sound compared with a normal tooth.

Pulp Vitality

The vitality of a tooth depends on the vascular supply to the tooth. However, most tests performed depend on neural responses. Because of the trauma disrupting the neurovascular bundle or immature root formation, the pulpal response to vitality testing may be widely variable immediately following a traumatic incident. The plexus of Raschkow is not completely developed in immature teeth, and the A-delta fibers that are responsible for the response to vitality tests do not mature until approximately 4 years after the tooth develops. However, testing should be done in all situations to have a baseline for future comparison.

Pulp vitality is tested by thermal tests and the electric pulp tester (EPT) (**Fig. 4**). Before testing a tooth, it should be dried and isolated properly to avoid false responses. The most common methods of cold testing use Endo-Ice, ethyl chloride spray, or sticks of ice. Sticks of ice may drip on the gingival and cause false-positive responses, and ethyl chloride spray is highly inflammable. Endo-Ice is sprayed onto a cotton pellet or cotton-wood stick and immediately applied to the tooth.

The response to the thermal test may be (1) no response, (2) mild-to-moderate transient pain response, (3) strong painful response that subsides quickly following

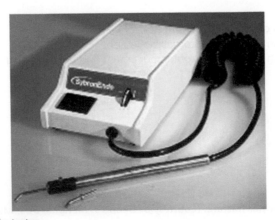

Fig. 4 Electric pulp tester.

removal of the stimulus, or (4) strong painful response that lingers for a period after removal of the stimulus.

The EPT stimulates the neural elements within the pulp and elicits a response. The test merely indicates whether the pulp is vital or necrotic; it does not provide information regarding the health or integrity of the pulp. The tooth is isolated and the electrode coated with a viscous conductor is placed on the middle one-third of the facial surface of the tooth. Any restoration should be avoided as it may cause a false reading. The current flow is adjusted to increase slowly, thus avoiding a painful experience for the patient. A complete circuit between the patient, the clinician, and the EPT should be maintained.

The vitality tests should be performed on adjacent and contralateral teeth for comparison. These tests are highly subjective and a definitive diagnosis is done using information that is gleaned from signs and symptoms, clinical and radiographic examination, and vitality tests.

Laser Doppler Flowmetry

Pulp vitality is most accurately assessed by the extent and condition of vascular supply. Tests that rely on the passage of light through a tooth for assessing vascular supply have been studied, as methods for detecting pulp vitality. One such test, laser Doppler flowmetry (LDF), is a noninvasive, objective, painless, semiquantitative method, using a laser light that is transmitted to the pulp by means of a fiberoptic probe. Scattered light from moving red blood cells (in a vital pulp) is reflected and returned by afferent fibers, producing a signal that helps in the differentiation of vital and necrotic pulp. A review of the relevant literature on LDF in the context of endodontics assessed its ability to estimate pulpal vitality in adults and children.[8] Although case reports have demonstrated vitality up to 6 months after tooth trauma,[9] assessments may be highly susceptible to environmental factors, technique-sensitive, and time-consuming. Nonpulpal signals, principally from periodontal blood flow, may contaminate the signal.[10] Currently LDF is not readily available for dental use.

SUMMARY

Complete chronologic documentation of the details of the traumatic incident, medical assessment, and dental assessment are crucial to successful management. Optimal care can only be provided to a traumatized patient after a comprehensive examination and assessment of the condition. A medical assessment of the patient can help the dental practitioner in identifying life-threatening or preexisting medical conditions that mandate medical referral. In this manner the dental practitioner is able to reduce the possibility of further complications and provide comprehensive dental assessment, treatment, and follow-up as needed.

REFERENCES

1. Andreasen JO, Andreasen FM, editors. Textbook and color atlas of traumatic injuries to the teeth. 3rd edition. St Louis (MO): Mosby; 1994.
2. Xiao WL, Zhang DZ, Wang YH. Aspiration of two permanent teeth during maxillofacial injuries. J Craniofac Surg 2009;20(2):558–60.
3. Teasdale G, Murray G, Parker L, et al. Adding up the Glasgow Coma Score. Acta Neurochir Suppl (Wien) 1979;28(1):13–6.
4. Ellis E 3rd, Scott K. Assessment of patients with facial fractures. Emerg Med Clin North Am 2000;18(3):411–48, vi [review].

5. Armstrong BD. Lacerations of the mouth. Emerg Med Clin North Am 2000;18(3): 471–80, vi [review].
6. da Silva AC, de Moraes M, Bastos EG, et al. Tooth fragment embedded in the lower lip after dental trauma: case reports. Dent Traumatol 2005;21(2):115–20.
7. Guidelines for the management of traumatic dental injuries—2007. International Association of Dental Traumatology. Available at: www.iadt-dentaltrauma.org. Accessed September 12, 2009.
8. Jafarzadeh H. Laser Doppler flowmetry in endodontics: a review. Int Endod J 2009;42(6):476–90.
9. Lee JY, Yanpiset K, Sigurdsson A, et al. Laser Doppler flowmetry for monitoring traumatized teeth. Dent Traumatol 2001;17(5):231–5.
10. Evans D, Reid J, Strang R, et al. A comparison of laser Doppler flowmetry with other methods of assessing the vitality of traumatized anterior teeth. Endod Dent Traumatol 1999;15(6):284–90.

Managing Injuries to the Primary Dentition

Dennis J. McTigue, DDS, MS

KEYWORDS

- Dental injuries • Primary teeth • Avulsion • Luxation
- Intrusion • Crown fractures • Root fractures

Dental injuries to preschool children can be challenging to manage because of the child's and parents' anxiety and the potential for damage to the developing permanent tooth buds. A conservative treatment approach that minimizes the potential emotional trauma to the child while prioritizing the healthy development of the permanent incisors is advised.

ETIOLOGY AND EPIDEMIOLOGY

Differences in study design and sampling criteria make it difficult to accurately determine the incidence and prevalence of traumatic injuries to the primary dentition. Reports indicate that 30% to 40% of preschool children suffer injuries to the primary dentition with the prevalence equal between boys and girls.[1,2] This probably underestimates the actual occurrence of trauma as many apparently minor injuries go unreported.

The teeth most commonly injured are the maxillary central incisors.[2,3] Predisposing factors include increased overjet and incompetent lip closure. Falls are the most common cause of injuries to young children particularly in the toddler stage as they develop mobility skills. A disturbing cause of oral injuries in children is child abuse. Up to 75% of all injures of abused children occur in the head and neck region.[4,5] Signs of abuse include tears of labial frena, injuries in various stages of healing, and injuries whose clinical presentation is inconsistent with the history provided by the caregiver.[6] Other signs include bruising of the labial sulcus in patients who are not walking, bruising of the soft tissues of the cheek or neck (accidental falls are more likely to bruise the forehead or chin), and human hand marks or pinch marks on the cheeks and ears.[7]

EXAMINATION AND DIAGNOSIS
History

A thorough medical and dental history is required to accurately diagnose the injured child's condition. The potential severity of the injury is determined by knowing

Division of Pediatric Dentistry, Ohio State University College of Dentistry, 305 W. 12th Avenue, Columbus, OH 43210, USA
E-mail address: mctigue.1@osu.edu

Dent Clin N Am 53 (2009) 627–638
doi:10.1016/j.cden.2009.07.002
0011-8532/09/$ – see front matter © 2009 Elsevier Inc. All rights reserved.

when, where, and how it occurred. The time elapsed since the injury affects the treatment and, most often, the prognosis. Knowledge of the mechanism of the injury helps determine its severity and the risk of associated injuries.

The child's medications and drug allergies should be determined with particular attention paid to immunizations. Tetanus prophylaxis is significant when the child suffers wounds that are contaminated by dirt as can occur with avulsions, intrusions, or deep lacerations. Reports indicate that increasing numbers of children in the United States are not getting appropriate immunizations because their parents believe that vaccinations are harmful or because of their growing cost. Children can achieve immediate passive immunity to tetanus with an injection of tetanus toxoid and tetanus immune globulin so any question about the adequacy of a child's tetanus protection should prompt a medical referral.[8]

Severe head injury should also be ruled out. If there is a history of loss of consciousness, confusion, vomiting, headache, personality change, nausea, seizure or disorientation, patients should be referred for immediate neurologic evaluation.[9–11]

Clinical Examination

It is essential that the clinician conduct a comprehensive and thorough extraoral and intraoral examination. Many clinicians find it helpful to use a trauma assessment form to record data and to organize the management of care (**Fig. 1**). An injured preschool child is frequently unable to cooperate and lay passively in a dental chair for the examination. In some cases a thorough examination can be obtained by using the knee-to-knee technique with the parent or an assistant (**Fig. 2**). On rare occasions it may be necessary to use techniques of protective stabilization using a restraining device (**Fig. 3**). Informed consent from the parent is required before protective stabilization is employed.[12]

Extraoral examination
All extraoral injuries to the head and neck region, including bruises, contusions, swelling, and lacerations, should be recorded. Facial bone fractures can be detected by careful palpation to determine discontinuities. Mandibular function and range of motion in all excursive movements should be checked. Neck stiffness or pain can signal cervical spine injury and immediate medical referral is indicated.

Intraoral examination
A soft-tissue examination should be completed to rule out lacerations and perforations. Careful attention should be paid to the presence of foreign bodies embedded in lacerated tissues as lack of thorough debridement can cause chronic infection and scarring.

Each tooth should be checked for mobility, fracture, and dislocation. Gently percussing each tooth is an excellent way to detect periodontal ligament (PDL) inflammation, though a frightened child provides an exaggerated response to any stimulus. For this reason, vitality tests are not routinely performed on primary teeth.

Radiographic examination
Radiographs are critical to an accurate diagnosis of an injured tooth. Films taken soon after an injury detect acute changes, such as dislocations, root fractures, foreign bodies, alveolar fractures and, possibly, injuries to developing permanent teeth. Follow-up radiographs taken at 3 to 4 weeks postinjury can help detect inflammatory root resorption, apical osteitis and calcific changes in the pulpal lumen.

Children's HOSPITAL

THE OHIO STATE UNIVERSITY

Trauma Form

Date of treatment _____
Doctor treating _____

Patient's Name _____
Medical Number _____
Age _____ yrs _____ mos
Sex □ male □ female
Race □ Cau □ Afr-Amer
□ Asian □ Native Amer

Date of Injury _____
Time Since Injury _____

Tetanus Concern □ No □ Yes
Date of Last Booster

How Injured □ Fall □ Hit □ MVA
□ Skateboard □ Other

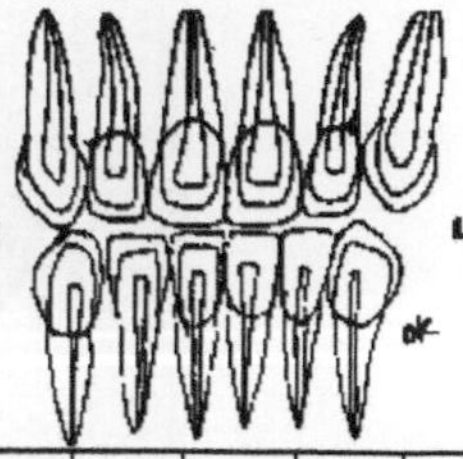

EXTRAORAL ASSESSMENT

CNS Status
_____ □ Normal
_____ □ Dizziness □ Seizure
_____ □ Headache □ Other
□ Unconscious □ Nausea

Hard Tissue
_____ □ Normal
_____ □ Infection □ Cranial Fx
_____ □ Mand Fx □ Max Fx
□ Zyg Fx

Soft Tissue
_____ □ Normal
_____ □ Laceration □ Abrasion
_____ □ Contusion □ Infection
□ Embedded Material
□ Swell □ Other

INTRAORAL ASSESSMENT

Hard Tissue
_____ □ Alveolar Fx □ Deglove
_____ Other _____

Soft Tissue
_____ □ Lips □ Tongue
_____ □ Buccal mucosa □ Frenum
□ Gingiva □ Palate

Dental Occlusion: □ Normal □ Abnormal

Classification: Molar _____ Cuspid _____
Overjet ____mm Overbite ____%
Openbite _____ X-bite _____

Jaw Opening: □ WNL □ Limited

Radiographs □ Periapical □ Occlusal
□ Lateral Anterior □ Panorex
□ Soft Tissue □ Lat Jaw Film
□ Other

Behavior problem □ Yes □ No

Radiograph Findings: _____
_____
_____
_____

R   L

Tooth No.					
Concussion					
Class I Fx					
Class II Fx					
Class III Fx					
Intrusion					
Extrusion					
Avulsion					
Subluxation					
Lateral luxation					
Root Fx					
Fragments					
Other					

Tooth No.					
Exposure					
Hemorrhage					
Heat					
Cold					
Contamination					
Vitalometer					
Percussion					
Mobility					

SUMMARY & DIAGNOSIS

Crown _____
Pulp _____
Root _____
Periapical _____

TREATMENT

Soft tissue □ Suture □ Other _____
Pulp □ Cvek □ Direct Pulp Cap
□ CaOH □ Formo □ Dycal
Restoration □ ZOE □ Composite
□ Ketac
Splinting □ No □ Yes, type _____

Medication □ Antibiotic _____
□ Analgesic _____
□ Other _____
Consult requested □ No □ Yes

RECALL FOLLOW-UP

□ 1 week □ 2 weeks □ 3 weeks
□ month □ 6 weeks □ 2 months
□ None □ Other _____

Fig. 1. Trauma assessment form.

The standard occlusal view is a simple and reliable exposure to detect injuries to anterior primary teeth (**Fig. 4**). In cases of multiple tooth injuries or suspected root fractures, additional occlusal views taken from slightly different horizontal angles can improve the accuracy of the diagnosis. A lateral anterior view can also be helpful to determine the relationship between an intruded primary incisor and its permanent successor, or to localize foreign bodies embedded in soft tissues (**Fig. 5**). Exposure times will vary according to the radiographic equipment used but doubling the exposure time is usually adequate for the lateral anterior film. A reduction to one third of the normal exposure time may be necessary to secure an adequate soft-tissue film.

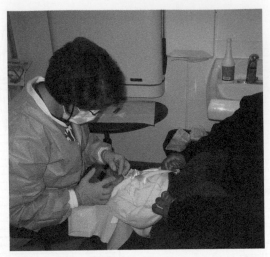

Fig. 2. Knee to knee examination technique.

TREATMENT

As noted earlier, the most important consideration in managing injured primary teeth should be the well being of the developing permanent successors. Parents should be thoroughly informed of the intimate relationship between the apex of the primary incisor and the developing permanent tooth bud. The benefits of saving an injured primary tooth versus the potential risk of damage to the developing permanent tooth should be explained and documented. This understanding is integral to acquiring valid informed consent from a distraught parent requesting heroic measures to save an injured primary tooth.

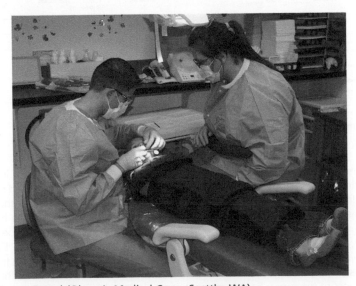

Fig. 3. Papoose Board (Olympic Medical Corp., Seattle, WA).

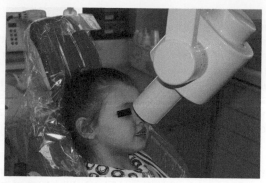

Fig. 4. Occlusal radiograph.

Luxation Injuries

Luxation injuries imply damage to the PDL and are the most common injuries in the primary dentition.[13] This frequency is because the supporting tissues in young children are pliable and allow the teeth to move, frequently without fracturing.

Concussion

A concussion injury transmits the force of the blow to the PDL but causes no mobility. The only clinical sign will be tenderness to percussion. Treatment is rarely needed, but adjusting the occlusion may relieve symptoms in a hypersensitive child. The concussed tooth should be monitored for several months to rule out potential complications.

Subluxation

The subluxed tooth has increased mobility but is not displaced from its socket. Sulcular bleeding may be present. Parents are instructed to keep the area clean and to have the child avoid incising on the involved teeth for 2 weeks. Subluxation is a common injury in the primary dentition and return to normal function occurs in the majority of cases, though close monitoring for pathologic sequelae is indicated.

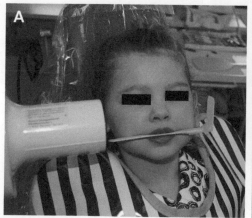
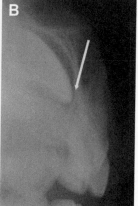

Fig. 5. Lateral anterior radiograph. (*A*) Clinical view. (*B*) Radiographic image demonstrating lack of contact between intruded primary incisor and the developing permanent successor (*arrow*).

Lateral luxation

This is a more serious injury with the tooth displaced out of its normal position, frequently in a palatal direction. Radiographs are indicated to rule out root fractures and to indicate the position of the root in the alveolus. If the tooth is not interfering with the occlusion it may be allowed to reposition spontaneously.[13] Some authors recommend that when occlusal interference does occur the tooth should be manually repositioned and splinted for 2 to 3 weeks.[14] Owing to the increased risk of pulpal necrosis and to the potential for damage to the developing permanent successor, however, this author recommends extracting severely displaced primary incisors.[15,16]

Intrusion

Intrusion of a primary incisor implies a high risk of damage to the permanent successor and the injured child's parents should be so advised at the time of injury.[17] Conservative treatment is indicated as damage to the permanent tooth bud can occur during extraction of the intruded primary incisor.[18] A lateral anterior radiograph (see Fig. 5) is taken to determine the position of the intruded primary incisor relative to the developing tooth bud. The majority of intruded incisors are displaced labially and away from the tooth bud (see Fig. 5B). These incisors are allowed to re-erupt spontaneously anticipating that most will survive without complications.[19] If the intruded tooth impinges on the developing tooth bud it is carefully extracted with the forceps gently engaged on the tooth's mesial and distal surfaces.[15] The great majority of intruded primary incisors will partially or completely re-erupt within 4 to 5 months (Fig. 6).[19,20]

Extrusion

The extruded tooth is displaced centrally from its socket and has increased mobility. Radiographs should be taken to rule out other injuries. Treatment is determined by the degree of extrusion, mobility, and the child's ability to cope with treatment. Minor extrusions can be repositioned, but severe extrusions should be extracted.[15]

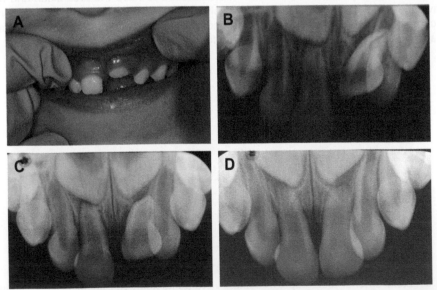

Fig. 6. Intruded primary incisor. (A) Day of injury. (B) Radiograph on day of injury. (C) 3 weeks postinjury. (D) 5 months postinjury.

Avulsion

Avulsed primary incisors should not be replanted because of the risk of damage to the permanent successors.[15,17,21,22] Radiographs are indicated to confirm that the tooth is not intruded. Losing anterior primary teeth is often more traumatic for the parents than it is for the injured child and the clinician must thoroughly explain the rationale against replantation. Once the primary canines have erupted, there is little concern about loss of space in the anterior segment with early loss of primary incisors.[23] If esthetics is a major concern, a fixed or removable partial denture can be fabricated (**Fig. 7**).

Crown Fractures

Any blow that causes a tooth to fracture is likely to also cause a luxation injury. The clinician is advised to carefully examine all fractured teeth and to manage associated luxation injuries as noted previously.

Uncomplicated crown fractures

These fractures include the enamel only, or enamel and dentin, but without a pulp exposure. Periapical radiographs are indicated to rule out other injuries and to assess the degree of physiologic root resorption. In minor fractures, the sharp edges can be smoothed with sandpaper disks or finishing burs. In larger fractures, including the incisal angle, adhesive resin-based composite restorations or preveneered stainless steel crowns may be indicated.[24]

Complicated crown fractures

These injuries involve a pulp exposure and treatment is predicated on the life expectancy of the tooth and the child's behavior (**Fig. 8**). In young children with immature

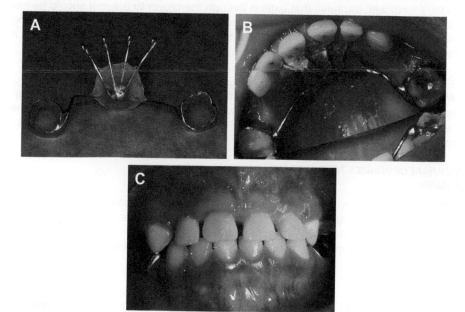

Fig. 7. Pediatric fixed partial denture. (*A*) Before placement of celluloid crown forms. (*B*) Immediate postinsertion demonstrating composite resin extruding from crown forms. (*C*) Facial view of finished appliance. (*Courtesy of* James W. Presich, Mishawaka, IN.)

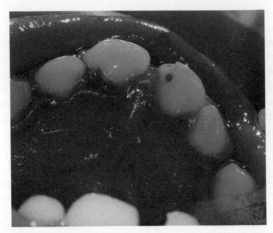

Fig. 8. Complicated crown fracture.

roots (less than 3 years) a pulpotomy is indicated to preserve the pulp vitality in the root.[25] When the root is mature, a complete pulpectomy with a resorbable paste, such as zinc oxide and eugenol, may be performed. Treatment of complicated crown fractures should be completed as soon as practical after the injury, usually within 1 or 2 days. As noted earlier, the child must be controlled to complete the pulpal therapy and to restore the tooth, often indicating sedation[26] or protective stabilization.[12] Parental informed consent is required for these management techniques.

Crown/Root Fractures

Primary teeth with fractures that extend through the crown to the root should be extracted. A radiograph is indicated to assess the degree of damage. To avoid injuring the developing tooth bud, root fragments should be left to resorb spontaneously if they cannot be extracted easily.[15]

Root Fractures

When primary roots fracture in the apical third, the coronal fragment may not be displaced and may have adequate stability to allow its retention in the mouth. If the coronal fragment is displaced it should be extracted and the apical fragment left to resorb spontaneously.[15]

SEQUELAE OF INJURIES TO THE PRIMARY DENTITION
Pulpitis

Pulpitis is the tooth's initial response to trauma and it accompanies almost every injury. Signs include sensitivity to percussion and capillary congestion that may be clinically apparent from the lingual surface of the tooth using transillumination. Pulpitis may be reversible in minor injuries or may progress to irreversible pulpitis and pulp necrosis.

Pulp Necrosis

Injured pulps may lose their vitality either because of damage to the vascular tissue at the apex and the resulting ischemia or because of necrosis of exposed coronal pulp tissue. If the necrotic pulp becomes infected with oral microorganisms, either caused by luxation of the root and ingress through the lacerated PDL or by way of an exposed pulp, pain and root resorption can occur. Once the inflammatory exudate vents to the oral cavity, usually through the thin labial alveolar plate, the condition becomes chronic and painless. Extraction is indicated to prevent damage to the permanent successor. The necrotic pulp may remain asymptomatic, clinically and radiographically, when it is not infected.

Tooth Discoloration

Injuries to the primary incisors frequently cause tooth discoloration (**Fig. 9**). Blood vessels within the pulp chamber can rupture depositing blood pigment in the dentinal tubules. This blood pigment may resorb completely or can persist to some degree throughout the life of the tooth. Teeth that discolor are not necessarily necrotic, particularly when the color change occurs within a few days of the injury. However, teeth with dark discoloration that persists for months after the injury are likely to be necrotic, but may remain asymptomatic.[27]

In healthy children, tooth color alone does not dictate treatment. Other signs or symptoms of infection, such as periapical radiolucency, pain, swelling, parulis, or increased mobility, should be detected before the tooth is extracted (see **Fig. 9**B).

Inflammatory Resorption

Inflammatory resorption can occur internally or externally. It is related to an infected pulp and an inflamed PDL. It can resorb roots quickly and the inflammatory process can damage developing teeth, so extraction of the offending tooth is indicated.

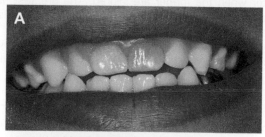
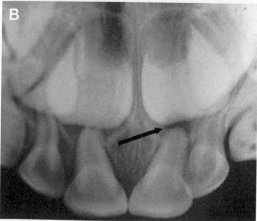

Fig. 9. Tooth discoloration. (*A*) Discolored primary incisor. (*B*) Periapical radiolucency (*arrow*).

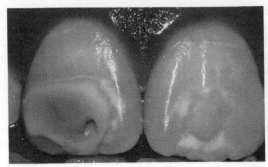

Fig. 10. Permanent incisors damaged secondary to trauma to their primary predecessors.

Pulp Canal Obliteration

Pulp canal obliteration is a common finding in luxated primary incisors, particularly when the injury occurred before completion of the tooth's root development. The entire pulp chamber and canal appear radiopaque in radiographs and the crown may have a yellowish color. The process of accelerated dentinal apposition in pulp canal obliteration is not well understood but these teeth tend to resorb normally and treatment is usually not indicated.[28]

Injuries to Developing Teeth

As noted throughout this article, the close proximity of the apices of primary incisors to the developing tooth buds of their permanent successors creates a potential for damage to the latter when the former are injured. The greatest risk for injuries to permanent teeth exists when the primary teeth are intruded or avulsed and before 3 years of age, when the permanent tooth crowns are calcifying.[17,29] White or yellow-brown discoloration is the most common deformity but enamel hypoplasia, crown and root dilacerations and ectopic or delayed eruption have all been reported (**Fig. 10**).[30,31]

SUMMARY

The management of injuries to the primary dentition is complicated by the child's age, ability to understand and cooperate for treatment, and by the potential for collateral damage to the developing permanent tooth buds. Clinicians treating children should be readily available after hours to provide care. Treatment priorities should include adequate pain control, safe management of the child's behavior, and protection of the developing permanent teeth.

REFERENCES

1. Glendor U. Epidemiology of traumatic dental injuries – a 12 year review of the literature. Dent Traumatol 2008;24(6):603–11.
2. Glendor U, Marcenes W, Andreasen JO. Classification, epidemiology and etiology. In: Andreasen JO, Andreasen FM, Andersson L, editors. Textbook and color atlas of traumatic injuries to the teeth. 4th edition. Oxford(UK): Blackwell Munksgaard; 2007. p. 224, 227.
3. Glendor U, Halling A, Andersson L, et al. Type of treatment and estimation of time spent on dental trauma. A longitudinal and retrospective study. Swed Dent J 1998;22:47–60.

4. da Fonseca M, Feigal R, ten Bensel R. Dental aspects of 1248 cases of child maltreatment on file at a major county hospital. Pediatr Dent 1992;14:152–7.
5. Maguire S, Junter B, Hunter L, et al. Diagnosing abuse: a systematic review of torn frenum and other intraoral injuries. Arch Dis Child 2007;92(12):1113–7.
6. American Academy of Pediatrics, American Academy of Pediatric Dentistry. Oral and dental aspects of child abuse and neglect. Pediatrics 1999;104:348–50.
7. Welbury RR, Murphy JM. The dental practitioner's role in protecting children from abuse. 2. The orofacial signs of abuse. Braz Dent J 1998;184(2):61–5.
8. American Academy of Pediatrics. Tetanus (Lockjaw). In: Pickering LK, editor. Red book: 2006 report of the Committee on Infectious Diseases. 27th edition. Elk Grove Village (IL): American Academy of Pediatrics; 2006. p. 648–53.
9. Tecklenburg F, Wright M. Minor head trauma in the pediatric patient. Pediatr Emerg Care 1991;7:40–7.
10. Johnston MV, Gerring JP. Head trauma and its sequelae. Pediatr Ann 1992;21: 362–8.
11. Da Dalt L, Marchi AG, Laudizi L, et al. Predictors of intracranial injuries in children after blunt head trauma. Eur J Pediatr 2006;165:142–8.
12. American Academy of Pediatric Dentistry. Guideline on behavior guidance for the pediatric dental patient. Pediatr Dent 2008;30(Suppl 7):125–33.
13. Borum MK, Andreasen JO. Sequelae of trauma to primary maxillary incisors. Part I. Complications in the primary dentition. Endod Dent Traumatol 1998;14:31–44.
14. Flores MT. Traumatic injuries in the primary dentition. Dent Traumatol 2002;18: 287–98.
15. Flores MT, Malmgren B, Andersson L, et al. Guidelines for the management of traumatic dental injuries. III. Primary teeth. Dent Traumatol 2007;23(4):196–202.
16. Soporowski NJ, Allred EN, Needleman HL. Luxation injuries of primary anterior teeth – prognosis and related correlates. Pediatr Dent 1994;16:96–101.
17. Assunção LR, Ferelle A, Iwakura ML, et al. Effects on permanent teeth after luxation injuries to the primary predecessors: a study in children assisted at an emergency service. Dent Traumatol 2009;25:165–70.
18. Flores MT, Holan G, Borum M, et al. Injuries to the primary dentition. In: Andreasen JO, Andreasen FM, Andersson L, editors. Textbook and color atlas of traumatic injuries to the teeth. 4th edition. Oxford (UK): Blackwell Munksgaard; 2007. p. 516–41.
19. Holan G, Ram D. Sequelae and prognosis of intruded primary incisors: a retrospective study. Pediatr Dent 1999;21:242–7.
20. Gondim JO, Moreira Neto JS. Evaluation of intruded primary incisors. Dent Traumatol 2005;21:131–3.
21. Andreasen JO, Ravn JJ. The effect of traumatic injuries to primary teeth on their permanent successors. II. A clinical and radiographic follow-up study of 213 injured teeth. Scand J Dent Res 1971;79:284–94.
22. Zamon EL, Kenny DJ. Replantation of avulsed primary incisors: a risk-benefit assessment. J Can Dent Assoc 2001;67:386–9.
23. Rock WP. Extraction of primary teeth – balance and compensation. In UK National clinical guidelines in paediatric dentistry. Int J Paediatr Dent 2002;12:151–3.
24. Waggoner WF. Restorative dentistry for the primary dentition. In: Pinkham J, Casamassimo P, Fields H, editors. Pediatric dentistry; infancy through adolescence. 4th edition. St. Louis (MO): Elsevier Saunders; 2005. p. 368–9.
25. Fuks AB. Pulp therapy for the primary dentition. In: Pinkham J, Casamassimo P, Fields H, et al, editors. Pediatric dentistry: infancy through adolescence. 4th edition. St. Louis (MO): Elsevier Saunders; 2005. p. 384–6.

26. American Academy of Pediatric Dentistry. Guideline for monitoring and management of pediatric patients during and after sedation for diagnostic and therapeutic procedures. Pediatr Dent 2008;30(Suppl 7):143–59.

27. Holan G, Fuks AB. The diagnostic value of eq4k-gray discoloration in primary teeth following traumatic injuries. Pediatr Dent 1996;18:224–7.

28. Jacobsen I, Sagnes G. Traumatized primary anterior teeth: prognosis related to calcific reactions in the pulp cavity. Acta Odontol Scand 1978;36:199.

29. Sennhenn-Kirchner S, Jacobs H. Traumatic injuries to the primary dentition and effects on the permanent successors – a clinical follow-up study. Dent Traumatol 2006;22:237–41.

30. Andreasen JO, Flores M. Injuries to developing teeth. In: Andreasen JO, Andreasen FM, Andersson L, editors. Textbook and color atlas of traumatic injuries to the teeth. 4th edition. Oxford (UK): Blackwell Munksgaard; 2007. p. 542–76.

31. Korf SF. The eruption of permanent central incisors following premature loss of their antecedents. J Dent Child 1965;32:39–44.

Minor Traumatic Injuries to the Permanent Dentition

Alex J. Moule, BDSc, PhD[a],*, Christopher A. Moule, BDSc[b]

KEYWORDS

- Dental trauma • Trauma to permanent dentition
- Crown and root fractures • Luxation injuries • Avulsion

Much literature discusses the causes and incidence of trauma to the dentition.[1–5] Although most injuries occur as a result of falls and play accidents,[6] an ever-increasing incidence of trauma from traffic accidents, sporting injuries, risk-taking activities, violence, and child physical abuse[7–9] has meant that managing dental trauma has become an important part of clinical dental practice. More than 20% of children experience damage to their permanent dentition by 14 years of age, with men outnumbering women 2:1, and peak incidence at 8 to 10 years of age.

Although single-tooth injuries are most common, motor vehicle and sporting injuries often involve damage to multiple teeth. Treatment is often distressing for patients and difficult for practitioners. Several studies discuss the adverse psychological consequences of dental trauma.[10] This article reviews the early management of traumatized permanent teeth, recommendations for which have been produced by the International Association of Dental Traumatology,[11,12] the American Academy of Pediatric Dentistry,[13] the American Association of Endodontists, and appear in numerous texts[1,5,8,14] and articles.[11,12]

Treatment invariably has two components: short-term emergency treatment and stabilization, and long-term endodontic management and review.[15] The classification of dental injuries described by Andreasen and colleagues[1] is generally followed.

ASSESSING TRAUMATIC DENTAL INJURIES IN PERMANENT TEETH

The systematic assessment of patients who have traumatic dental injuries is well covered in the literature.[1,5,14] Emphasis has also been placed on the need for an interdisciplinary approach to management and to record a detailed and thorough history, not only to document the specific circumstances surrounding the incident but also to provide an accurate record for legal and insurance reporting.[14] In this respect, all

[a] School of Dentistry, University of Queensland c/o A. Moule, 9th Floor, 141 Queen Street, Brisbane 4000, Queensland, Australia
[b] 1 Adelaide Park Road, Yeppoon 4703, Queensland, Australia
* Corresponding author.
E-mail address: alex@endodonticsonly.com (A.J. Moule).

Dent Clin N Am 53 (2009) 639–659
doi:10.1016/j.cden.2009.06.004
0011-8532/09/$ – see front matter © 2009 Elsevier Inc. All rights reserved.

dental injuries should be meticulously documented and supported by appropriate sketches or photographs. Test results should be accurately recorded so reports can be written and future comparisons can be made.

Although this article addresses only the examination and management of the local dental injuries, clinicians must recognize that some dental injuries may not be accidental in nature. Injuries must be assessed vigilantly to distinguish, when possible, between accidental injuries and those resulting from abuse.[7–9,16]

SOFT TISSUE MANAGEMENT

Hard tissue injuries also often involve damage to the supporting structures. When this occurs, the prognosis for the tooth (particularly with respect to the vitality of the pulp) is poorer.[17] Any examination must include assessment of both components. Soft tissue injuries should be assessed; displaced or lacerated tissues immediately repositioned; and, where necessary, these should be sutured into place (**Fig. 1**).[1] When lacerations occur concomitantly with tooth fractures, tissues should be examined radiographically for the presence of embedded tooth fragments and debris (**Fig. 2**).

BITE TESTING

In general, if a patient can close their teeth together firmly without hurting, any fracture of the jaw or joint damage is unlikely. If the patient cannot close together firmly, the injury must be assessed to determine whether the jaw is fractured or teeth have been displaced, or both. Similarly, if a patient can open widely and simultaneously move their jaw from side to side without discomfort, any joint damage is unlikely. Pain on jaw movement must be examined closely and appropriate radiographs taken to exclude bone and joint damage.

PERCUSSION SENSITIVITY, PERCUSSION TONE, AND MOBILITY

Teeth that are sensitive to percussion have experienced damage to the supporting tissues. If they exhibit a lower tone than normal when percussed, they have usually been extruded or loosened in their socket. Teeth that exhibit higher tone immediately after trauma are often wedged into the bone.[14] Mobility implies loosening of the tooth within the socket. Mobility of several teeth or groups of teeth indicates an associated alveolar fracture or a fracture of the alveolar plate. Thus, in examining tooth mobility,

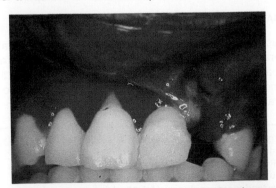

Fig. 1. Displaced soft tissues must be immediately repositioned and sutured into place. Lack of attention to soft tissues in this case has resulted in a disfiguring gingival defect, a painful healing process, and poorer prognosis for injured teeth (*Courtesy of* G Heithersay AO, BDS, MDS, DDSc, Brisbane, Queensland, Australia).

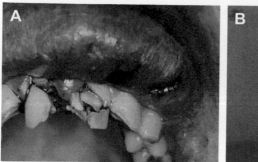
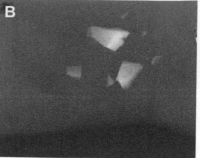

Fig. 2. When tooth structure loss occurs in association with lacerations, soft tissues must be examined clinically (A) and radiographically (B) for the presence of tooth fragments in tissues.

teeth should be examined individually and teeth and groups of teeth tested against each other.

In adults, tenderness to percussion with concussed and subluxated teeth can take time (months) to settle. No emergency treatment is required except judicious grinding to free the tooth from occlusion. Prolonged sensitivity to percussion can also occur as a result of small fractures in the alveolar plate (**Fig. 3**A). These teeth need splinting. Pulp extirpation will not relieve these symptoms (see **Fig. 3**B).

PULP SENSIBILITY TESTING

Response to cold testing is the most reliable and accurate way of testing teeth in children.[16] Routine sensibility testing of the traumatized and adjacent teeth should occur as soon as possible after injury, and then at regular intervals, to form a baseline for

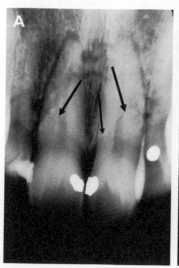
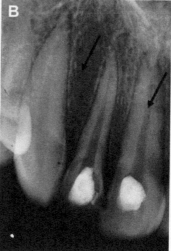

Fig. 3. (A) Continued sensitivity to biting on teeth that have sustained concussion injuries may be caused by fractures of the buccal alveolar plate (arrow). (B) Pulp extirpation in these teeth, as has occurred, is unwarranted and will not relieve the sensitivity.

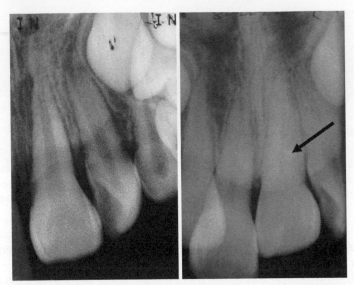

Fig. 4. Pulp testing procedures only measure neural response. Lack of response to testing does not imply that the pulp is irreversibly damaged. The presence of hard tissue changes (*arrow*) occurring in the pulp chamber is a clear indication that the pulp tissue is vital.

future comparisons. Because sensibility results can be unpredictable immediately after trauma, initial testing may be delayed for a short time after injury, particularly in the presence of hemorrhage and associated soft tissue injuries, or when sensitivity to thermal stimulation or touching the exposed surface clearly indicates that the pulp is responsive.

Longer observation times ($\geq$8 weeks initially) may be required before a definitive decision can be made regarding the state of the pulp.[18,19] Pulp tests only measure neural response and do not assess pulp vitality, which is dependant on blood supply. Damage to neural structures can often occur without damage to the more flexible vascular elements. Thus, although many traumatized teeth may not respond to sensibility testing, progressive radiographic changes in pulpal anatomy can show that the pulp is healthy (**Fig. 4**). Reversals of negative sensibility testing results can occur, particularly in immature teeth and teeth with open apices. Of particular clinical

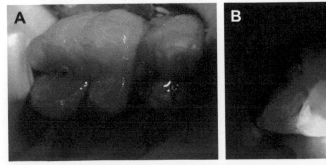

Fig. 5. Transillumination using a bright light source of this otherwise intact mandibular molar (*A*) subjected to severe indirect force in a car accident shows multiple cracks and enamel infractions (*B*).

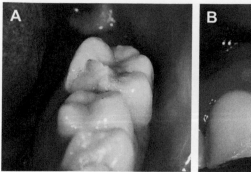
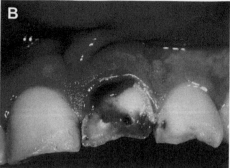

Fig. 6. Indirect trauma resulting from the mandibular and maxillary teeth being forcibly brought together can result in widespread cracking and fracture of molar teeth (*A*), the importance of which is sometimes underestimated in assessing dental injuries. In this type of injury, incisor subgingival fractures are often located labially (*B*). Although the left incisor is obviously damaged, the right has sustained a deep anterior labial subgingival fracture (*arrow*).

importance are teeth that exhibit reversals in responses from positive to negative. Pulps in these teeth have most probably become necrotic. Necrosis will generally occur within the first 6 months of injury.

TRANSILLUMINATION

Using a bright light to assess for enamel cracks and detect subtle changes in color, which may not otherwise be obvious, is invaluable.[16] Transillumination also helps to identify traumatized teeth that do not show obvious signs of trauma (**Fig. 5**).

TYPE OF FORCE

An assessment of the type of force or blow that caused the trauma is sometimes overlooked. Factors to consider include the type of trauma (direct or indirect), the composition (soft, hard, resiliency) and speed of the object, the direction of the blow, and whether teeth came into contact with objects or the ground.

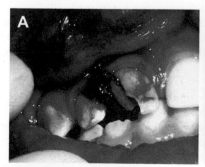
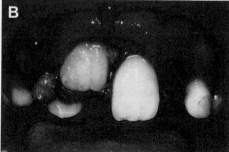

Fig. 7. (*A*) A small hard object trauma, in this case a stone, caused a severe localized dental injury. (*B*) A larger soft object injury caused widespread dental injuries involving displacement of soft tissues, intrusion, luxation, and avulsion of teeth and bone fractures (*Courtesy of* Richard Widmer, BDSc, MDSc, Sydney, NSW, Australia).

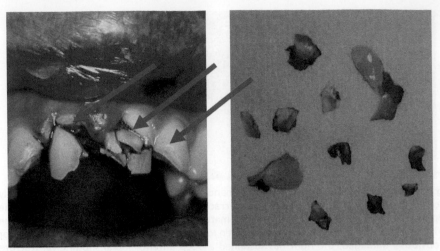

Fig. 8. Assessing the direction of the impacting force and the size of the object can help determine the extent of the injuries.

With indirect trauma, the upper and lower teeth are forcibly brought together. If the energy of impact is great, widespread damage occurs, often resulting in significant damage (including deep subgingival fractures) to molar teeth (**Fig. 6**A). These injuries are difficult to manage. Subgingival crown–root fractures in anterior teeth from indirect trauma are usually labially subgingival (see **Fig. 6**B).

The damage occasioned to the teeth and surrounding tissues is influenced by the composition and resiliency of the impacting object. Impact with hard objects (eg, stones) results in localized site-specific injuries, with penetrating soft tissue injuries and tooth fractures in an area corresponding to the size of the object (**Fig. 7**A). The extent of the injury is usually obvious.

The severity of the injury is directly related to the size and weight and speed of the object. Injuries that are accompanied by tooth fractures do not always result in severe damage to supporting structures or the pulp, because some of the energy of impact is absorbed by the fracture.

Resilient objects often cause more widespread injury, including displacement of soft tissues, luxation and avulsion of teeth, and bony fractures (see **Fig. 7**B). The extent of the injury is less obvious and more widespread examination is required.

The direction of the impacting blow can be helpful in visualizing the extent of the injury. Dental injuries are situated distal (or away from) the point of first contact and depend on the direction of the impacting force (**Fig. 8**). This assessment is sometimes helpful in legal reporting.

RADIOGRAPHIC EXAMINATION

All teeth affected by the injury must be examined radiographically to ascertain the severity of the trauma, the stage of root development, injuries to the supporting structures, and the presence of root fractures. At least one "straight on" view is required for each tooth. When root fractures are suspected, several angulations are required. When supporting tissues and/or joint injuries are suspected, an orthopantomogram image is essential. Cone beam imaging is helpful for assessing intrusive injuries, bony fractures, and resorption.[20–22]

PREVIOUS DENTAL TRAUMA

Patients often experience injuries to teeth on several occasions, as is commonly seen in patients who have a large overjet and incompetent lips. Whether any injured teeth have been previously traumatized is important to establish, because this can complicate diagnosis and influence prognosis.

THE MANAGEMENT OF CRACKED AND FRACTURED TEETH
Infraction

Infraction involves cracking of the enamel without loss of tooth structure, and is best seen with transillumination. Pulpal complications are rare (0%–3.5%) unless an associated luxation injury is present.[1,23,24] No emergency treatment is necessary. Pulp treatment is unnecessary unless signs of irreversible pulpitis or pulp necrosis are present. Pulp sensibility testing should be performed after 3 and 12 months, and radiography performed at 12 months to assess intrapulpal calcification.

Uncomplicated Crown Fractures

In uncomplicated crown fractures, tooth structure is lost without exposure of the pulp. Pulpal complications rarely occur where only enamel is fractured (0%–1%),[24–26] unless an associated luxation injury is present (8.5%).[25] When both enamel and dentine are involved, pulpal complications are also infrequent (0%–6%),[27–29] unless a concomitant luxation injury is present, wherein the incidence of necrosis can be as high as 25%.[27,28]

Factors influencing pulp survival include type and site of fracture, presence of a luxation injury, type of treatment undertaken, and timing of treatment. Pulp necrosis occurs more often in deep angular fractures and deep fractures that remain untreated for more than 24 hours. Thus, dentine should be covered as soon as possible.

Lost tooth structure can be restored with restorative materials[1,11,30] or through re-attaching the fragment.[1,11,31–33] Fragment reattachment can be a simple and very effective procedure with good longevity (**Fig. 9**).[34] Therefore, patients should be advised to bring fragments (and teeth) with them when presenting for treatment. Pulps can become necrotic several years after injury. Routine testing should be undertaken at to 8 weeks and then at yearly intervals.[35]

Complicated Crown Fractures

Complicated fractures are those in which the pulp is exposed. In the absence of an associated luxation injury, pulp necrosis does not usually occur immediately, although

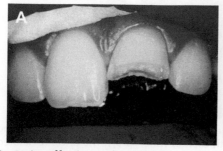 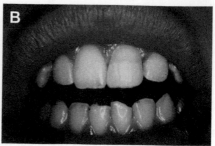

Fig. 9. An effective and predictable way to restore a fractured anterior tooth (*A*) is to reattach the crown fragment (*B*) (*Courtesy of* Peter Greer, BDSc, MDSc, Brisbane, Queensland, Australia).

this is the inevitable outcome if exposed pulps remain untreated. Except in immature teeth,[36,37] most traumatically exposed pulps will become necrotic and infected if left untreated for 1 month.[38] Recommended treatment procedures include pulp capping, partial pulpotomy, pulpotomy, and pulpectomy.

In young patients in whom root development is not complete, the goal of treatment is to maintain pulp vitality to allow closure of the root apex and promote root development. Preferred treatment consists of using partial pulpotomy procedures,[39] removing a portion of the pulp (2–3 mm) with a gentle technique (high-speed diamond bur with copious water spray), eliminating blood clots (using irrigation), and capping with calcium hydroxide or mineral trioxide aggregate (MTA) (**Fig. 10**).[40–42]

Proponents of MTA highlight that, although success rates are similar to those with calcium hydroxide, its placement is easier, it sets, it can act as a permanent restoration with a superior seal, it is unlikely to dissolve away, and it does not have to be removed later. Medicaments must be placed directly onto healthy noninflamed tissue, and the site then protected against bacteria. Regular review (at 6–8 weeks and then yearly) is recommended to assess pulp vitality and continued root development.

Although root therapy is often considered preferred treatment for mature teeth with closed apices, partial pulpotomy techniques can be useful for all traumatically fractured teeth, regardless of patient age and degree of apical closure of the teeth.[43] This can represent considerable practical and economic advantages. Definitive restorations can be placed immediately, avoiding problems associated with temporary restoration breakdown and reinoculation of the exposure site with bacteria. The fragment can be reattached before or after root canal treatment or partial pulpotomy where possible.[1,11,31–33]

Crown–root Fractures

Crown–root fractures involve enamel, dentine, and the root surface, and usually pass subgingivally. The pulp is often exposed. Factors that influence treatment planning include position and circumferential extent of the fracture, severity of the fracture in a subgingival direction, root maturity, and pulp exposure. Treatment options reviewed by Heithersay and Moule[44] include periodontal surgery to expose crown margins;

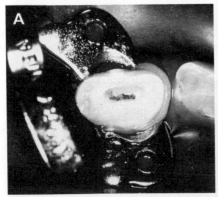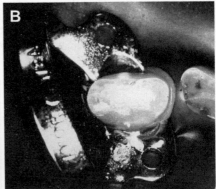

Fig. 10. Cvek pulpotomy. (*A*) The pulp chamber is accessed to a level of 2 to 3 mm using a gentle technique (high-speed round bur with copious water spray). The uncontaminated pulp is irrigated. When bleeding ceases, calcium hydroxide or mineral trioxide aggregate is placed onto the pulp (*B*) and the tooth restored with a leak-proof restorative material (*Courtesy of* David Cable, BDS, MDSc, Sydney, NSW, Australia).

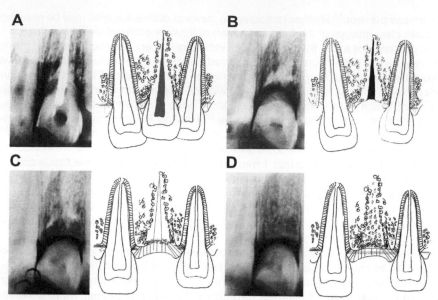

Fig. 11. Surgical root submergence is a treatment option for submerging ankylosed teeth in young patients or for teeth with deep subgingival fractures. (*From* Malmgren B, Malmgren O, Andreasen JO. Alveolar bone development after decoronation of ankylosed teeth. Endod Top 2006;14:35–40; with permission.)

reattachment of the fragment; restorative management only with extension of margins of the restoration below the level of the gingival margin; orthodontic extrusion; intentional replantation; surgical repositioning; autotransplantation; root submergence; extraction and replacement; and orthodontic space closure. Although treatment of crown–root fractures can be complex and time consuming, many teeth can be predictably retained.[13,44] Implant replacement is a viable alternative in adult patients who have severe fractures.

In younger patients, treatment priority should be development of the root rather than restoration of aesthetics and function. Dressing an exposed pulp and restoring lost tooth structure with a temporary denture is sometimes better until the root matures and restoration is practical. Reattaching the fragment (before or after pulp therapy) can stabilize the crown until the tooth erupts, bringing the subgingival margin into a more favorable position, sometimes without the need for further intervention, or until the patient reaches an age at which more definitive treatment is practical.

When a tooth is deemed unrestorable in a growing patient, decoronation (**Fig. 11**) may be indicated to preserve bone.[45,46] This procedure allows normal alveolar development before implant placement when growth is complete,[47–49] and preserves labio-palatal width, which may negate the need for ridge augmentation procedures.[16]

Root Fractures

Root fractures usually occur in a horizontal or oblique direction, and in a subgingival or infrabony position. Although they can present without clinical signs of crown displacement, the crown is usually extruded and lingually displaced. The radiographic appearance is influenced by the position of the fracture and the direction of the beam. Fractures can be single or multiple and appear radiographically as single or multiple lines across the root.[50] Multiple radiographic views at different angles may be required to obtain clear images of the fracture. A high oblique or occlusal view is useful.[11]

The presence of a root fracture is not an indication for endodontic treatment; this is only required if pulp necrosis has occurred.[51] Many root-fractured teeth survive without treatment. Pulp survival rates are higher in root-fractured teeth than in traumatized teeth without fracture. Many heal without intervention in one of three modalities: hard tissue interposition; interposition of bone and periodontal ligament; and interposition of periodontal ligament alone.[52] Healing is more favorable in incompletely formed teeth and when displacement of the coronal fragment is minimal.[52] The occurrence of pulp necrosis is significantly higher if the fragments are separated more than 1 mm (suggesting that 1 mm is the limit to which the pulpal tissue can be stretched before the neural and vascular components become compromised).[52] Calcification of the pulp canal, often erroneously called "pulp canal obliteration," is a common feature that may develop in root-fractured teeth. This condition is rarely a problem in the long-term and can only develop if tissues in the pulp maintain their vitality.

A nonhealing inflammatory process associated with pulp necrosis and infection of the coronal fragment can also occur. The probability of this occurring is affected by apical maturation, location of the fracture, extent of dislocation, and separation between the fragments. If necrosis develops (20%–44% of cases),[52] it is generally detectable after 2 to 5 months. Invariably, only the coronal fragment becomes necrotic as the blood supply to the apical fragment remains intact.[51]

Responses to thermal and electrical tests immediately after trauma are an unreliable means of predicting final outcomes.[53,54] Diagnosis of pulp status occurs later and is based on development of radiolucency at the fracture site and presence of a sinus or coronal discoloration. Resorption apically or at the fracture site does not indicate necrosis.

Root fractures rarely occur in immature teeth; these teeth are more likely to be luxated or avulsed. Root fractures in immature teeth are often irregular and have a vertical and horizontal component. As the pulp is large and developmentally active, calcific healing usually occurs without the need for any intervention.

Appropriate treatment for root fractured teeth is assessed in two stages: at initial presentation to determine communication, displacement, and mobility, and several months later to assess pulp status mobility and healing of root-fractured teeth.

Initial presentation

If the fracture line is communicating with the oral cavity, the coronal fragment is removed and the remaining tooth structure treated on its merits. If the fracture line is not communicating with the oral cavity, the coronal fragment is assessed for displacement and mobility. If the fragment is mobile or displaced, it should be splinted immediately. Early and accurate repositioning reduces the likelihood of pulp necrosis.[55,56] Radiographic confirmation of the accuracy of repositioning is helpful. Splinting should be non-rigid, atraumatically placed and removed after 4 weeks, except in teeth that have fracture occurring in the coronal third, which may need splinting for up to 4 months.[35,55]

If the fracture does not communicate with the gingiva and is not mobile or displaced, no treatment is necessary. Endodontic management is not part of the initial treatment of root-fractured teeth. Percussion-sensitive root-fractured teeth can be splinted to alleviate symptoms. Pulp removal from a percussion-sensitive, vital root-fractured tooth will not generally relieve discomfort.

Later assessment

Unless symptoms dictate, assessment of the pulp status and healing of root-fractured teeth can be delayed for several months. Important considerations at this review appointment are pulp vitality and tooth mobility.

If signs of pulp necrosis and infection (radiographic evidence of bone loss at the fracture site, development of a sinus or tooth discoloration) are present, the pulp is removed down to the fracture site and apexification procedures involving the use of calcium hydroxide[52] and/or MTA[5,57] are instituted. Initial endodontic procedures should not extend beyond the fracture line. If the tooth remains mobile, long-term splinting is considered. In the absence of mobility or pulp necrosis, no treatment is undertaken.

Follow-up radiographs should be taken at 1 month, 2 months, and 6 months, and then at yearly intervals.[36]

THE MANAGEMENT OF LUXATION INJURIES

Luxated teeth have been moved bodily in relation to their supporting structures. Andreasen and colleagues[1] identified five types of luxation injury. Several studies have investigated the prognosis for these injuries.[58–62] Factors affecting prognosis are degree and type of displacement, treatment delays, root maturation, associated crown fractures, and emergency treatment provided. Long-term complications include pulp necrosis with infection, pulp canal calcification, ankylosis, and root resorption.

Luxation injuries result in a much higher incidence of pulp necrosis than injuries involving fractures of the teeth. Although most cases of pulp necrosis develop within 4 months, pulps can become necrotic and infected many years later. When assessing prognosis, the bulk of the pulp at the apex and how far the root apex has traveled in relation to its neurovascular support are important to consider. Bulky pulps in immature teeth can stretch and compress further before severing neural and vascular communications than can thinner pulps in more mature teeth. Root resorption, particularly in immature teeth, can develop and progress very rapidly. Thus, frequent short-term follow-up is essential, although long-term follow-up is also necessary.

Except for some intrusive injuries in mature teeth (and some avulsed mature teeth with long dry times), priority should be given to soft tissue repositioning and splinting before endodontic procedures are undertaken. Endodontic therapy should be commenced immediately when evidence of pulp necrosis or root resorption is present. Although immature teeth can revascularize and continue root development (evident radiographically), treatment should not be delayed in teeth that show any sign of root resorption, because inflammatory root resorption can occur rapidly and significant root structure can be lost in a matter of a week or two.

A noninfected apical remodeling process (transient apical breakdown) can occur. This entity can mimic pulp necrosis radiographically and in clinical observations. Andreasen[63] identified this uncommon process in 4.2% of luxated teeth. All showed resorptive widening of the apical foramen after injury, and most showed periapical radiolucency and color (often pinkish) or electrometric sensibility changes. Signs and symptoms later returned to normal.

Transient apical breakdown is more common in mild luxation injuries in fully formed, or almost fully formed, teeth (**Fig 12**). Recognition of this process is important to prevent unnecessary endodontic treatment. Transient apical breakdown may be more common than reported, because many patients may not present for treatment after mild luxation. A case can be made for observing asymptomatic teeth with early

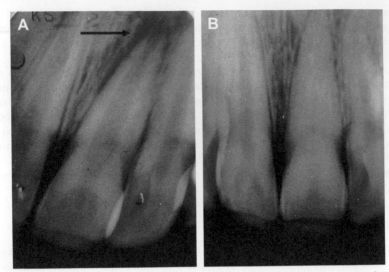

Fig. 12. Radiographs showing an example of transient apical breakdown. The first radiograph (*A*) shows evidence of widening of the apical foramen and apical breakdown, and a periapical lesion is present (*arrow*). In the second radiograph (*B*), the periapical radiolucency has resolved and the pulp has calcified, indicating recovery of the pulp.

signs of pulp necrosis in selected patients, but only when clinicians are confident they will be compliant with recall regimes. Continued root development and canal calcification indicates pulp vitality, even in the absence of responses to pulp sensibility testing. Regular radiographic examination is necessary (6–12 monthly). Endodontic therapy is commenced at the first radiographic or clinical evidence of pulp necrosis with infection (eg, symptoms, sinus formation, or darkening of the crown).

Concussion

Concussed teeth are characterized by a marked tenderness to percussion, but no abnormal loosening or displacement. Pulp necrosis (3%) or pulp canal obliteration (2%–7%) are infrequent complications.[14,64] Concussed teeth seldom show evidence of root resorption. No emergency treatment is required.

Subluxation

Subluxated teeth are characterized by abnormal loosening without displacement. These teeth are tender to percussion, and some bleeding in the gingival crevice may occur. Prognosis is good. Pulp necrosis occurs in 6% to 17% of teeth, canal calcification in 9% to 12%, and progressive root resorption in fewer than 2%.[14,64] Endodontic management is sometimes necessary, but only later when symptoms dictate.[64] Apart from judicious grinding to free the occlusion, no emergency treatment is required.

Extrusive Luxation

These teeth are extruded apically from their sockets, and minimal damage to the socket wall occurs. Pulp necrosis has been reported in 43% of teeth (usually within 12 months), pulp canal calcification in 35%, and progressive root resorption in

5.5%.[65] A direct correlation exists between degree of extrusion and incidence of pulp canal calcification, but not with necrosis.[65]

Extruded teeth should be immediately repositioned and splinted with a flexible splint for 2 to 3 weeks.[35,66] If complete repositioning is not possible because of treatment delay, arrangements may be required to reposition them further using gentle orthodontic forces. Radiographic examination and pulp sensibility testing is carried out at 2 weeks, 1 month, 2 months, 6 months, 12 months, and then yearly for several years.[35] Endodontic therapy is commenced immediately (particularly in immature teeth) if evidence of pulp necrosis with infection or root resorption is present.

Lateral Luxation

These teeth are displaced laterally in the socket. This dental injury is severe because it is accompanied by fracture or comminution of the socket wall. Teeth can be firmly locked into position and may require force to reposition them. Pulp necrosis (40% in children[67] and 58% in adults[64]), pulp canal calcification (40%),[67] and root resorption (26%)[64] are commonly reported sequelae. All laterally luxated teeth should be disimpacted, repositioned, and splinted into place as soon a possible. Delayed repositioning leaves the root surface in contact with bone, which influences the onset of root resorption. Teeth should be splinted for 4 weeks to allow healing of the alveolar fracture.[35] Endodontic therapy is often necessary. Pulp necrosis is influenced by root maturity and the distance the root apex moves in relation to the socket.

Intrusive Luxation

Intrusively luxated teeth are forcefully intruded into bone. Many are also associated with crown fractures.[68] Almost all mature intruded teeth become necrotic.[69-71] Progressive root resorption occurs in nearly 50% of cases. Delayed repositioning influences the onset of replacement resorption. Necrotic pulps should be removed to help prevent the onset of inflammatory root resorption.[12,72] Immediate (surgical) repositioning, splinting (4 weeks), and early pulp removal is preferred treatment for mature intruded teeth in adults.

Although orthodontic repositioning is another option,[73] intruded mature teeth are often so firmly wedged into the bone that normal orthodontic forces cannot disimpact them, and attempted orthodontic movement can result in the intrusion of adjacent teeth. Surgical repositioning is also a useful technique for multiple intruded teeth when orthodontic anchorage may be an issue. Care must be taken when repositioning teeth to ensure that the bone is brought down with teeth and that the soft tissues are sutured firmly into place.

In immature teeth, the apex is open and the bone is softer and more malleable. Because immature intruded teeth can spontaneously reposition themselves, resulting in significantly better healing, experts suggest delaying treatment for these teeth.[73] However, root resorption occurs in a large number of cases and careful monitoring is essential to ensure that this is detected and treated early.[69,70] If spontaneous repositioning does not seem to be occurring predictably, immature teeth should be brought down through orthodontic or surgical means as soon as possible after trauma. Some experts advocate disimpacting intruded immature teeth to assist with re-eruption.

Regular radiographic follow-up at 2 weeks, 1 month, 2 months, 6 months, and yearly is essential because root resorption can occur rapidly in immature teeth.[35] If resorption is detected, pulpectomy and treatment with calcium hydroxide (or a corticosteroid/antibiotic paste[74]) should be performed immediately.

Surgical exposure of the intruded immature teeth to permit endodontic therapy has been proposed.[75] The extent of intrusion and the presence of associated crown fractures are important prognostic considerations. Pulps in immature teeth seem to survive if the intrusion is less than 3 mm, whereas only 45% of these pulps survive if the intrusion is greater than 6 mm.[70] Almost all surviving intruded immature teeth undergo pulp canal calcification. Pulp necrosis is usually diagnosed within 6 months, but may develop years later in open-apex teeth.[69,70]

MANAGEMENT OF AVULSION INJURIES

Although the prognosis for an avulsed tooth must be guarded, replantation as soon as possible followed by a brief period of flexible splinting and endodontic therapy has been shown to be the most effective method of treatment. Vitality of the periodontal ligament cells is the critical factor affecting prognosis of replanted teeth. The shortest extra-oral period (<15 minutes), minimum manipulation of the tooth surface and socket, and use of an appropriate storage medium have been identified as factors that minimize root resorption.[76–79] The following factors are important to consider when treating avulsed teeth.

Extra-oral Dry Time

Extra-oral dry time and the stage of root development are the most critical factors associated with root resorption.[76,80] Teeth replanted immediately have the best long-term prognosis and the least incidence of root resorption. A relationship exists between the total area of root surface when the cells have become necrotic and the amount of replacement resorption generated.[75]

Contamination of the Root Surface

Contamination of the root surface is a prognostic indicator for root resorption.[80] Thus, teeth should be cleaned before replantation. However, rinsing in tap water should be avoided if possible.

Storage Medium

Storage in a suitable storage medium is critical if teeth cannot be replanted immediately. Acceptable solutions are milk, contact lens solution,[81] Hanks' Balanced Salt Solution, and saliva.[82,83] If a suitable storage solution is unavailable or teeth cannot be replaced immediately, wrapping in polyethylene film can be beneficial. Storage in tap water should be avoided.

Splinting

Splints should be flexible and used for a short time,[66] unless associated bony fractures necessitate longer splinting times. Longer splinting times (>10 days) and inflexible splints tend to promote resorption.[84,85]

Socket Preparation

Although gentle irrigation of the socket is recommended to remove any blood clots before replantation, curettage of the socket is not necessary.[12]

Tetanus Booster

It is important to ensure all patients are up to date with tetanus immunization.

Antibiotic Therapy

Systemic administration of antibiotics is generally recommended to prevent the harmful effects of bacterial contamination, although evidence supporting this is limited.[1,86,87] Applying topical doxycycline and minocycline to the root surface before replantation has been found to increase the chance of pulp revascularization and decrease the incidence of inflammatory root resorption and ankylosis in animals.[88,89] Immediate placement of an intracanal antibiotic and corticosteroid in mature teeth after replantation seems to prevent the development and progression of inflammatory root resorption,[74] although replacement resorption still occurs to some extent.[72]

Effect of Endodontic Therapy

In mature teeth, pulps should be extirpated as soon as possible[72] or after initial periodontal healing has occurred (at least within 7–10 days).[12,35,90] However, experts recommend delaying further endodontic therapy until an initial period of soft tissue healing has occurred.[1]

Stage of Root Development

Replantation of avulsed teeth with immature root development has been reviewed.[91] Because pulps in these teeth may survive, delaying endodontic treatment is recommended (in teeth with short extra-oral times only) to establish whether root formation continues. Revascularization seems inversely proportional to root length. Calcific changes within the pulp canal imply that the pulp has remained (or become) viable after the injury.

Care should be taken when delaying treatment if patient compliance cannot be assured. Regular clinical and radiographic examinations at short intervals (weeks) are recommended in these teeth to expeditiously identify inflammatory resorption, which progresses rapidly in immature tooth roots. If this is detected, immediate pulp extirpation, followed by intracanal medication, should be commenced.[74] Long-term treatment with calcium hydroxide has been questioned because of possible detrimental effects on the strength of the remaining root.[92,93] Revascularization of necrotic open apex teeth using polyantibiotic pastes is possible.[94]

Age of the Patient and Orthodontic Therapy

Although it is generally accepted that avulsed teeth should be replanted as soon as possible, the desirability of replanting contaminated avulsed teeth with long dry times in young patients about to enter a growth spurt has been questioned, particularly if orthodontic treatment is anticipated in the near future. Experts have suggested that, because all patients will experience ankylosis and replacement resorption over time, resulting in root submergence and compromised orthodontic treatment, immature teeth with long dry times should not be replanted. Andreasen and colleagues.[95] (citing issues relating to problems in selecting alternative treatments at surgery, chances of healing, psychological considerations, and concerns about preserving alveolar bone) propose that avulsed teeth in young children should be replanted irrespective of most extra-oral conditions. Alternatives to replantation include orthodontic closure and autotransplantation.[96]

Replantation is not as much of a problem in adult patients because the teeth are fully erupted and do not need to be moved into place. The periodontal ligament can be removed manually or through soaking in sodium hypochlorite before replantation. Treatment of the root surface with sodium fluoride has been advocated to inhibit the resorptive process.[1] Endodontic therapy for teeth with long dry times can be performed before or after replantation.

FOLLOW-UP

Radiographs should be taken at regular intervals of 1, 3, 6, and 12 months, and then regularly up to 10 years after avulsion.[35] Ankylosis-related tooth submergence should be monitored and treatment (extraction or surgical decoronation) instituted in younger patients if the tooth submerges more than 3 mm.

PRIORITIZING TREATMENT

Most dental injuries involve damage to one or two teeth.[16] However, often multiple teeth are injured and injuries are associated with soft tissue and alveolar fractures. In these cases, treatment must be prioritized and preference given to injuries for which time is important in determining long-term prognosis. Injuries that require early and immediate treatment (avulsions, extrusions, luxation injuries, displaced root fractures, soft tissues injuries, and alveolar fractures) must be treated sequentially and preferentially. Splinting procedures depend on the major injury.

Undisplaced root fractures, intrusions, and complicated crown fractures should be treated as soon as possible, but a short delay in treatment does not seem to affect prognosis. Treatment of crown fractures without pulp exposure can be delayed if circumstances prevent their early management. Early coverage of the dentine within 24 hours is recommended, particularly in deep corner fractures.

All teeth should be repositioned so that they are comfortable in occlusion. Judicious grinding should be performed to free the injured teeth from occlusion. Clinicians occasionally encounter teeth that have been poorly splinted into place during emergency treatment. Removing splints even a few days after an accident, repositioning the teeth, and then splinting them more suitably is often a simple procedure.

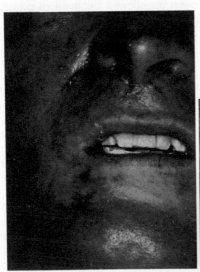
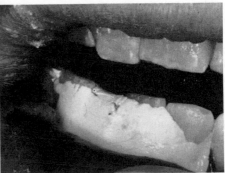

Fig. 13. When soft tissue injuries or medical problems prevent the management of painful, shattered, or mobile teeth, a periodontal pack can provide temporary stabilization of the teeth for a week or two and allow patients to function comfortably during that time.

Pain relief can be a priority. When major soft tissue injuries occur in association with fragmented teeth, sometimes removing fragments and splinting teeth immediately is not possible. When this occurs, pain can be relieved by stabilizing fragmented teeth and splinting mobile teeth with a standard periodontal pack, which can remain in place until soft tissue healing allows better access to the dentition (**Fig. 13**).

REFERENCES

1. Andreasen JO, Andreasen FM, Andersson L. Textbook and color atlas of traumatic injuries to the teeth. 4th edition. Oxford: Blackwell Munksgaard; 2007.
2. Caldas AF Jr, Burgos ME. A retrospective study of traumatic dental injuries in a Brazilian dental trauma clinic. Dent Traumatol 2001;17(6):250–3.
3. Skaare AB, Jacobsen I. Dental injuries in Norwegians aged 7–18 years. Dent Traumatol 2003;19(2):67–71.
4. Tapias MA, Jimenez-Garcia R, Lamas F, et al. Prevalence of traumatic crown fractures to permanent incisors in a childhood population: Mostoles, Spain. Dent Traumatol 2003;19(3):119–22.
5. Cohen S, Hargreaves KM. Pathways of the pulp. 9th edition. St. Louis (MO); London: Elsevier Mosby; 2006.
6. Hall RK. Pediatric orofacial medicine and pathology. 1st edition. London; Melbourne: Chapman & Hall Medical; 1994.
7. DiScala C, Sege R, Li G, et al. Child abuse and unintentional injuries: a 10-year retrospective. Arch Pediatr Adolesc Med 2000;154(1):16–22.
8. Welbury R, Wilson NHF, Whitworth JM, et al. Managing dental trauma in practice. London; Chicago: Quintessence Pub.; 2006.
9. Jessee SA. Continuing education: child abuse and neglect: implications for the dental profession. J Contemp Dent Pract 2003;4(2):92.
10. Fakhruddin KS, Lawrence HP, Kenny DJ, et al. Impact of treated and untreated dental injuries on the quality of life of Ontario school children. Dent Traumatol 2008;24(3):309–13.
11. Flores MT, Andersson L, Andreasen JO, et al. Guidelines for the management of traumatic dental injuries. I. Fractures and luxations of permanent teeth. Dent Traumatol 2007;23(2):66–71.
12. Flores MT, Andersson L, Andreasen JO, et al. Guidelines for the management of traumatic dental injuries. II. Avulsion of permanent teeth. Dent Traumatol 2007; 23(3):130–6.
13. Guideline on management of acute dental trauma. Pediatr Dent 2005;27(7 Reference Manual):135–42.
14. Andreasen JO. Traumatic dental injuries: a manual. 2nd edition. Oxford; Malden (MA): Blackwell Munksgaard; 2003.
15. Moule AJ, Moule CA. The endodontic management of traumatized permanent anterior teeth: a review. Aust Dent J 2007;52(1 Suppl):S122–37.
16. Cameron AC, Widmer RP, Australasian Academy of Paediatric Dentistry. Handbook of pediatric dentistry. 3rd edition. Edinburgh: Mosby Elsevier; 2008.
17. Andreasen FM. Pulpal healing after luxation injuries and root fracture in the permanent dentition. Endod Dent Traumatol 1989;5(3):111–31.
18. Jacobsen I. Criteria for diagnosis of pulp necrosis in traumatized permanent incisors. Scand J Dent Res 1980;88(4):306–12.
19. Andreasen FM. Transient root resorption after dental trauma: the clinician's dilemma. J Esthet Restor Dent 2003;15(12):80–92.

20. Cohenca N, Simon JH, Mathur A, et al. Clinical indications for digital imaging in dento-alveolar trauma. Part 2: root resorption. Dent Traumatol 2007;23(2):105–13.
21. Cohenca N, Simon JH, Roges R, et al. Clinical indications for digital imaging in dento-alveolar trauma. Part 1: traumatic injuries. Dent Traumatol 2007;23(2): 95–104.
22. Tsukiboshi M. Optimal use of photography and microcomputed tomography scanning in the management of traumatized teeth. Endod Top 2006;14:4–19.
23. Ravn JJ. Follow-up study of permanent incisors with enamel cracks as result of an acute trauma. Scand J Dent Res 1981;89(2):117–23.
24. Stalhane I, Hedegard B. Traumatized permanent teeth in children aged 7–15 years. Sven Tandlak Tidskr 1975;68(5):157–69.
25. Ravn JJ. Follow-up study of permanent incisors with enamel fractures as a result of an acute trauma. Scand J Dent Res 1981;89(3):213–7.
26. Robertson A. A retrospective evaluation of patients with uncomplicated crown fractures and luxation injuries. Endod Dent Traumatol 1998;14(6):245–56.
27. Ravn JJ. Follow-up study of permanent incisors with enamel-dentin fractures after acute trauma. Scand J Dent Res 1981;89(5):355–65.
28. Robertson A, Andreasen FM, Andreasen JO, et al. Long-term prognosis of crown-fractured permanent incisors. The effect of stage of root development and associated luxation injury. Int J Paediatr Dent 2000;10(3):191–9.
29. Zadik D, Chosack A, Eidelman E. The prognosis of traumatized permanent anterior teeth with fracture of the enamel and dentin. Oral Surg Oral Med Oral Pathol 1979;47(2):173–5.
30. Vitale MC, Caprioglio C, Martignone A, et al. Combined technique with polyethylene fibers and composite resins in restoration of traumatized anterior teeth. Dent Traumatol 2004;20(3):172–7.
31. Olsburgh S, Jacoby T, Krejci I. Crown fractures in the permanent dentition: pulpal and restorative considerations. Dent Traumatol 2002;18(3):103–15.
32. Maia EA, Baratieri LN, de Andrada MA, et al. Tooth fragment reattachment: fundamentals of the technique and two case reports. Quintessence Int 2003; 34(2):99–107.
33. Chu FC, Yim TM, Wei SH. Clinical considerations for reattachment of tooth fragments. Quintessence Int 2000;31(6):385–91.
34. Andreasen FM, Noren JG, Andreasen JO, et al. Long-term survival of fragment bonding in the treatment of fractured crowns: a multicenter clinical study. Quintessence Int 1995;26(10):669–81.
35. Traumatology IAoD. Available at: http://www.iadt-dentaltrauma.org. Accessed February 14, 2007.
36. Caliskan MK, Oztop F, Caliskan G. Histological evaluation of teeth with hyperplastic pulpitis caused by trauma or caries: case reports. Int Endod J 2003; 36(1):64–70.
37. Caliskan MK, Sepetcioglu F. Partial pulpotomy in crown-fractured permanent incisor with hyperplastic pulpitis: a case report. Endod Dent Traumatol 1993; 9(4):171–3.
38. AL-Nazhan S, Andreasen JO, AL-Bawardi S, et al. Evaluation of the effect of delayed management of traumatized permanent teeth. J Endodon 1995:391–3.
39. Cvek M. A clinical report on partial pulpotomy and capping with calcium hydroxide in permanent incisors with complicated crown fracture. J Endod 1978;4(8):232–7.
40. Karabucak B, Li D, Lim J, et al. Vital pulp therapy with mineral trioxide aggregate. Dent Traumatol 2005;21(4):240–3.

41. Chacko V, Kurikose S. Human pulpal response to mineral trioxide aggregate (MTA): a histologic study. J Clin Pediatr Dent 2006;30(3):203–9.
42. Witherspoon DE, Small JC, Harris GZ. Mineral trioxide aggregate pulpotomies: a case series outcomes assessment. J Am Dent Assoc 2006;137(5):610–8.
43. Blanco L, Cohen S. Treatment of crown fractures with exposed pulps. J Calif Dent Assoc 2002: 419–25.
44. Heithersay GS, Moule AJ. Anterior subgingival fractures: a review of treatment alternatives. Aust Dent J 1982;27(6):368–76.
45. Malmgren B. Decoronation: how, why, and when? J Calif Dent Assoc 2000;28(11): 846–54.
46. Malmgren B, Cvek M, Lundberg M, et al. Surgical treatment of ankylosed and infrapositioned reimplanted incisors in adolescents. Scand J Dent Res 1984;92(5): 391–9.
47. Filippi A, Pohl Y, von Arx T. Decoronation of an ankylosed tooth for preservation of alveolar bone prior to implant placement. Dent Traumatol 2001;17(2):93–5.
48. Schwartz-Arad D, Levin L, Ashkenazi M. Treatment options of untreatable traumatized anterior maxillary teeth for future use of dental implantation. Implant Dent 2004;13(1):11–9.
49. Malmgren B. Alveolar bone development after decoronation of ankylosed teeth. Endod Top 2006;14:35–40.
50. Andreasen JO, Hjorting-Hansen E. Intraalveolar root fractures: radiographic and histologic study of 50 cases. J Oral Surg 1967;25(5):414–26.
51. Cvek M, Mejare I, Andreasen JO. Conservative endodontic treatment of teeth fractured in the middle or apical part of the root. Dent Traumatol 2004;20(5): 261–9.
52. Andreasen JO, Andreasen FM, Mejare I, et al. Healing of 400 intra-alveolar root fractures. 1. Effect of pre-injury and injury factors such as sex, age, stage of root development, fracture type, location of fracture and severity of dislocation. Dent Traumatol 2004;20(4):192–202.
53. Lee JY, Yanpiset K, Sigurdsson A, et al. Laser Doppler flowmetry for monitoring traumatized teeth. Dent Traumatol 2001;17(5):231–5.
54. Bakland LK, Andreasen JO. Examination of the dentally traumatized patient. W V Dent J 1996;70(2):10–7.
55. Andreasen JO, Andreasen FM, Mejare I, et al. Healing of 400 intra-alveolar root fractures. 2. Effect of treatment factors such as treatment delay, repositioning, splinting type and period and antibiotics. Dent Traumatol 2004;20(4):203–11.
56. Bramante CM, Menezes R, Moraes IG, et al. Use of MTA and intracanal post reinforcement in a horizontally fractured tooth: a case report. Dent Traumatol 2006; 22(5):275–8.
57. Karabucak B, Li D, Lim J. Vital pulp therapy with mineral trioxide aggregate. Dent Traumatol 2005;21(4):240–3.
58. Humphrey JM, Kenny DJ, Barrett EJ. Clinical outcomes for permanent incisor luxations in a pediatric population. Dent Traumatol 2003:266–73.
59. Crona-Larsson G, Bjarnason S, Noren JG. Effect of luxation injuries on permanent teeth. Endod Dent Traumatol 1991;7(5):199–206.
60. Lee R, Barrett EJ, Kenny DJ. Clinical outcomes for permanent incisor luxations in a pediatric population. Dent Traumatol 2003:274–9.
61. Nikoui M, Kenny DJ, Barrett EJ. Clinical outcomes for permanent incisor luxations in a pediatric population. Dent Traumatol 2003:280–5.
62. Andreasen JO, Vinding TR, Christensen SSA. Predictors for healing complications in the permanent dentition after trauma. Endod Top 2006;14:20–7.

63. Andreasen FM. Transient apical breakdown and its relation to color and sensibility changes after luxation injuries to teeth. Dent Traumatol 1986;2(1):9–19.
64. Andreasen FM, Pedersen BV. Prognosis of luxated permanent teeth—the development of pulp necrosis. Endod Dent Traumatol 1985;1(6):207–20.
65. Lee R, Barrett EJ, Kenny DJ. Clinical outcomes for permanent incisor luxations in a pediatric population. II. Extrusions. Dent Traumatol 2003;19(5):274–9.
66. Kahler B, Heithersay GS. An evidence-based appraisal of splinting luxated, avulsed and root-fractured teeth. Dent Traumatol 2008;24(1):2–10.
67. Nikoui M, Kenny DJ, Barrett EJ. Clinical outcomes for permanent incisor luxations in a pediatric population. III. Lateral luxations. Dent Traumatol 2003;19(5):280–5.
68. Andreasen JO, Bakland LK, Matras RC, et al. Traumatic intrusion of permanent teeth. Part 1. An epidemiological study of 216 intruded permanent teeth. Dent Traumatol 2006;22(2):83–9.
69. Andreasen JO, Bakland LK, Andreasen FM. Traumatic intrusion of permanent teeth. Part 2. A clinical study of the effect of preinjury and injury factors, such as sex, age, stage of root development, tooth location, and extent of injury including number of intruded teeth on 140 intruded permanent teeth. Dent Traumatol 2006;22(2):90–8.
70. Humphrey JM, Kenny DJ, Barrett EJ. Clinical outcomes for permanent incisor luxations in a pediatric population. I. Intrusions. Dent Traumatol 2003;19(5):266–73.
71. Andreasen JO. Challenges in clinical dental traumatology. Endod Dent Traumatol 1985;1(2):45–55.
72. Bryson EC, Levin L, Banchs F, et al. Effect of immediate intracanal placement of Ledermix Paste(R) on healing of replanted dog teeth after extended dry times. Dent Traumatol 2002;18(6):316–21.
73. Andreasen JO, Bakland LK, Andreasen FM. Traumatic intrusion of permanent teeth. Part 3. A clinical study of the effect of treatment variables such as treatment delay, method of repositioning, type of splint, length of splinting and antibiotics on 140 teeth. Dent Traumatol 2006;22(2):99–111.
74. Chen H, Teixeira FB, Ritter AL, et al. The effect of intracanal anti-inflammatory medicaments on external root resorption of replanted dog teeth after extended extra-oral dry time. Dent Traumatol 2008;24(1):74–8.
75. Cvek M. Endodontic management of traumatized teeth. In: Andreasen JO, editor. Textbook and color atlas of traumatic injuries to the teeth. 3rd edition. Copenhagen: Mosby; 1994. p. 598–647.
76. Andreasen JO, Borum MK, Jacobsen HL, et al. Replantation of 400 avulsed permanent incisors. 4. Factors related to periodontal ligament healing. Endod Dent Traumatol 1995;11(2):76–89.
77. Andreasen JO, Borum MK, Andreasen FM. Replantation of 400 avulsed permanent incisors. 3. Factors related to root growth. Endod Dent Traumatol 1995;11(2):69–75.
78. Andreasen JO, Borum MK, Jacobsen HL, et al. Replantation of 400 avulsed permanent incisors. 2. Factors related to pulpal healing. Endod Dent Traumatol 1995;11(2):59–68.
79. Andreasen JO, Borum MK, Jacobsen HL, et al. Replantation of 400 avulsed permanent incisors. 1. Diagnosis of healing complications. Endod Dent Traumatol 1995;11(2):51–8.
80. Kinirons MJ, Gregg TA, Welbury RR, et al. Variations in the presenting and treatment features in reimplanted permanent incisors in children and their effect on the prevalence of root resorption. Br Dent J 2000;189(5):263–6.

81. Al-Nazhan S, Al-Nasser A. Viability of human periodontal ligament fibroblasts in tissue culture after exposure to different contact lens solutions. J Contemp Dent Pract 2006;7(4):37–44.
82. Sigalas E, Regan JD, Kramer PR, et al. Survival of human periodontal ligament cells in media proposed for transport of avulsed teeth. Dent Traumatol 2004; 20(1):21–8.
83. Andreasen JO. Effect of extra-alveolar period and storage media upon periodontal and pulpal healing after replantation of mature permanent incisors in monkeys. Int J Oral Surg 1981;10(1):43–53.
84. Andersson L, Lindskog S, Blomlof L, et al. Effect of masticatory stimulation on dentoalveolar ankylosis after experimental tooth replantation. Endod Dent Traumatol 1985;1(1):13–6.
85. Oikarinen K. Tooth splinting: a review of the literature and consideration of the versatility of a wire-composite splint. Endod Dent Traumatol 1990;6(6):237–50.
86. Hammarstrom L, Blomlof L, Feiglin B, et al. Replantation of teeth and antibiotic treatment. Endod Dent Traumatol 1986;2(2):51–7.
87. Andreasen JO, Jensen SS, Sae-Lim V. The role of antibiotics in preventing healing complications after traumatic dental injuries;a literature review. Endod Top 2006; 14:80–92.
88. Ritter AL, Ritter AV, Murrah V, et al. Pulp revascularization of replanted immature dog teeth after treatment with minocycline and doxycycline assessed by laser Doppler flowmetry, radiography, and histology. Dent Traumatol 2004;20(2):75–84.
89. Cvek M, Cleaton-Jones P, Austin J, et al. Effect of topical application of doxycycline on pulp revascularization and periodontal healing in reimplanted monkey incisors. Endod Dent Traumatol 1990;6(4):170–6.
90. Finucane D, Kinirons MJ. External inflammatory and replacement resorption of luxated, and avulsed replanted permanent incisors: a review and case presentation. Dent Traumatol 2003;19(3):170–4.
91. Johnson WT, Goodrich JL, James GA. Replantation of avulsed teeth with immature root development. Oral Surg Oral Med Oral Pathol 1985;60(4):420–7.
92. Andreasen JO, Munksgaard EC, Bakland LK. Comparison of fracture resistance in root canals of immature sheep teeth after filling with calcium hydroxide or MTA. Dent Traumatol 2006;22(3):154–6.
93. Andreasen JO, Farik B, Munksgaard EC. Long-term calcium hydroxide as a root canal dressing may increase risk of root fracture. Dent Traumatol 2002;18(3): 134–7.
94. Banchs F, Trope M. Revascularization of immature permanent teeth with apical periodontitis: new treatment protocol? J Endod 2004;30(4):196–200.
95. Andreasen JO, Malmgren B, Bakland LK. Tooth avulsion in children: to replant or not. Endod Top 2006;14:28–34.
96. Stenvik A, Zachrisson BU. Missing anterior teeth: orthodontic closure and transplantation as viable options to conventional replacements. Endod Top 2006;14: 41–50.

Revisiting Traumatic Pulpal Exposure: Materials, Management Principles, and Techniques

Leif K. Bakland, DDS*

KEYWORDS

- Dental trauma • Crown fractures • Vital pulp therapy
- Pulpotomy

Vital pulp therapy has a long history in dentistry.[1,2] Its purpose is to maintain vitality of the pulp, a goal that is particularly desirable in the case of young, immature teeth (**Fig. 1**). The use of vital pulp therapy is, however, not necessarily confined to developing teeth; any tooth, regardless of stage of development and maturity, can be preserved after traumatic or accidental exposure if the pulp is healthy. It is now also recognized that many teeth with carious pulp exposure can have vital pulp therapy with predictable outcomes.[3] Success depends on a good understanding of pulp biology, the use of appropriate materials, and sound technical procedures.

This article presents current concepts of managing teeth with traumatic pulp exposures. The article includes a description of the traumatology of crown fractures, discussion of treatment considerations, a summary of materials for vital pulp therapy, and an outline of techniques for treating pulp exposures.

TRAUMATOLOGY OF CROWN FRACTURES

Crown fractures are common traumatic injuries to teeth[4] and are categorized as enamel fractures, uncomplicated fractures (enamel-dentin fractures), complicated fractures (involving enamel, dentin, and exposure of the pulp), and crown-root fractures, which may be uncomplicated (no pulpal involvement) or complicated (with pulpal involvement).

Department of Endodontics, School of Dentistry, Loma Linda University, Loma Linda, CA 92350, USA
* Corresponding author.
E-mail address: lbakland@llu.edu

Dent Clin N Am 53 (2009) 661–673
doi:10.1016/j.cden.2009.06.006
0011-8532/09/$ – see front matter

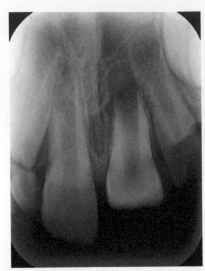

Fig.1. Radiograph of fractured left maxillary central incisor in a boy, age 6. Failure to protect the exposed pulp will lead to pulp necrosis and stop root development. Even though endodontic apexification in such a tooth can be done, the tooth will be weak and subject to cervical root fracture. Also, recognize that the radiolucent area surrounding the apex is normal in a developing tooth and does not indicate an apical lesion. (*Courtesy of* Leif K. Bakland, DDS, Loma Linda, CA.)

A crown fracture that involves dentin exposes the pulp whether one can see and touch the soft pulp tissue or not. This is because a fracture involving dentin exposes dentinal tubules in direct communication with the pulp. Therefore, in crown fractures without direct pulp exposure in the teeth of young patients, it is prudent to protect the exposed dentin to prevent bacterial toxins, which are generated from the biofilm that quickly covers the surface of a fractured tooth, from penetrating through the exposed dentinal tubules into the pulp. The closer the fracture is to the pulp and the younger the patient, the larger is the diameter of the dentinal tubules.

A complicating factor associated with crown fractures is that the trauma may concomitantly have caused a luxation injury to the tooth, compromising the ability of the pulp to defend itself and recover from the injury. Luxation injuries damage the supporting structures, such as the periodontal ligament and the neurovascular bundle supplying the pulp through the apical foramen. If bacteria gain access to the pulp, either directly through a traumatic exposure or through open dentinal tubules, and the pulp is compromised because of reduced or cut-off blood supply, the pulp will likely become necrotic.

TREATMENT CONSIDERATIONS

Treatment of an uncomplicated crown fracture can today be accomplished quite successfully by either a build-up with acid-etched composite resin or by reattaching the broken segment, if available, using a bonding system (**Fig. 2**). The expected outcome for either approach is excellent: nearly 100% pulp survival regardless of root developmental status.[5] Timely protection of exposed dentin in young, developing teeth is advisable to prevent the pulp from undergoing infection-related necrosis.

Complicated crown fractures in which direct pulp exposure occurs should not be viewed as hopeless situations for pulp survival (**Fig. 3**).[6] Correctly managed, many

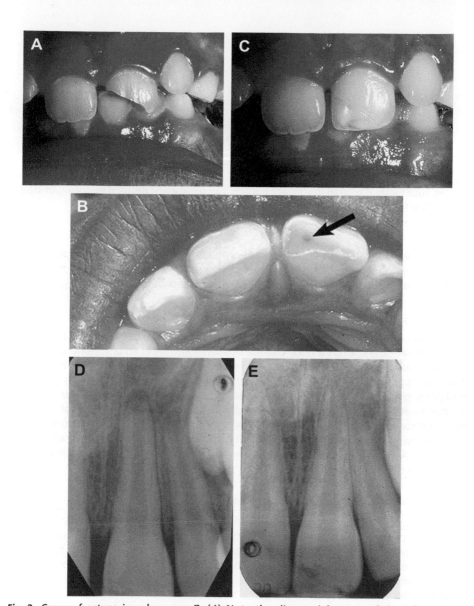

Fig. 2. Crown fracture in a boy, age 7. (*A*) Note the diagonal fracture of the left central incisor. (*B*) Arrow points to where the pulp can be seen close to the fracture site. (*C*) The broken tooth fragment was rebonded to the tooth, an excellent way to protect the pulp when it is close to the fracture surface. (*D*) Radiograph shows the tooth immediately after the rebonding procedure. Note the wide-open apex and thin root walls. (*E*) Radiograph taken 2 years posttrauma. The pulp remained vital and the root continued to mature, as can be seen by comparing the two central incisors. (*Courtesy of* Todd Milledge, Loma Linda, CA.)

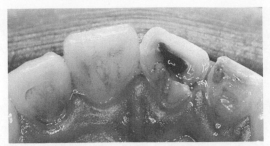

Fig. 3. Complicated crown fracture with exposed pulp. With today's materials and techniques, such teeth, if treated in a timely fashion, can survive and develop mature root structures. (*Courtesy of* Leif K. Bakland, DDS, Loma Linda, CA.)

teeth can be treated using relatively simple procedures to allow continued pulpal function, an important consideration in young, immature teeth. Before any treatment approach is chosen, however, a number of questions should be asked.

First: How Long Ago was the Accident?

A common notion among many dentists is that if a pulp has been exposed for more than 24 to 48 hours, it has a poor chance of surviving. This is an unfortunate misconception that has led to unnecessary pulp removal of vital, productive pulp that could have been preserved. Like tissue from other kinds of wounds, exposed pulp soon develops granulation tissue to protect the exposed wound surface. True enough, bacteria will invade the pulp tissue gradually, but it can take many days for bacteria to penetrate even a few millimeters.[7] Cvek[6] demonstrated that the pulpotomy technique known by his name could successfully be done even several days after pulp exposure. A good rule is to proceed as soon as possible, but as long as the pulp is alive it can be treated.

Second: What is the Stage of Tooth Development?

If the fracture occurs in an adult with a fully formed root, and the treatment plan includes a prosthetic crown, it is probably more practical to perform the endodontic treatment prior to restoring the tooth because it would be undesirable to later have to do root canal treatment through a prosthetic crown. If, however, the tooth can be restored either by placing a composite resin build-up or by reattaching the fractured segment, the tooth can receive the same vital pulp therapy as recommended when developing teeth in young patients are fractured, which will be described below.

With respect to patient age and stage of tooth development, it is very important to make every effort to preserve pulp vitality in young patients with still developing teeth. Continued pulp vitality facilitates continued root development.[8] This is a concept often overlooked when dealing with crown fractures. Practitioners tend to look at the root apex and, if that looks closed or nearly so, the assumption is that the tooth is fully formed. The area of the root that should be examined closely on the radiograph is the cervical part of the root. Young developing teeth often lack root thickness and that needs to develop even if the apical opening appears closed. Continued root development can be expected if the exposed pulp is properly protected. Vital pulp therapy, to be described below, is the goal in the management of crown fractures with pulp exposure in young patients.

Third: How Much Tooth Structure Remains?

Extensive loss of coronal tooth structure complicates the management of crown fractures. In cases involving both the crowns and the roots of teeth in adults, it often is prudent to consider extraction and replacement with an implant or a bridge. However, in young patients still growing and developing, efforts to save the injured teeth should be made even if the treatment is complex. In some cases, even if eventual loss is likely, it is worth saving the teeth for as long as possible in order to maintain the ridge contour, particularly in the maxillary anterior region.[9]

In addition to determining the extent of damage, one should ask if the broken crown fragment is available. Particularly in young patients, reattaching a fractured crown fragment can be a very satisfactory approach to restoration of the tooth (See **Fig. 2**). The current-generation bonding agents provide an excellent means of reattaching the fragments to the remaining tooth. Resistance to refracture, while not equal to normal teeth, is quite acceptable.[10,11]

While reattachment of fractured tooth fragments has become very acceptable in children, it is not often done in adults. There is, however, no technical reason why this procedure cannot also be done in adults. It may be that esthetic considerations, however, will dictate restoration with a porcelain veneer or a prosthetic crown.

Fourth: How Large is the Pulp Exposure?

This is a question that has relatively little importance.[12] If the pulp is to be preserved, the exposure needs only to be small enough to accommodate bridging with a restorative material. A healthy pulp, regardless of how much tissue is exposed, has a great ability to survive as long as it can be protected from bacteria.

MATERIALS FOR VITAL PULP THERAPY

Many dental materials have been proposed for protecting exposed dental pulps: calcium hydroxide, hydrophilic resins, resin-modified glass ionomer, tricalcium phosphate, and mineral trioxide aggregate (MTA).[3] Are some materials better than others? It is probably safe to say that a dental material per se has little direct effect on pulp tissue, particularly after the material has set into its permanent stage. The reason some materials do better than others when placed on exposed pulps relate to the ability of the individual material to prevent bacterial contamination of the pulp. This was clearly demonstrated by Cox and colleagues.[13] The most important characteristic then of a dental material with respect to its value in vital pulp therapy is its ability to prevent microleakage.

The best known and most widely used vital pulp therapy material has for many years been calcium hydroxide. First used over 80 years ago[1] in teeth with deep carious lesions, calcium hydroxide in time became recognized as a valuable pulp-capping and pulpotomy material. In modern times, perhaps no one has done more to promote the use of calcium hydroxide than Miomir Cvek, a pediatric dentist in Stockholm, Sweden, who was both a researcher and a clinician. His technique has been known as the *Cvek pulpotomy technique* and probably many thousands of teeth have been saved by the technique he promoted (**Fig 4**).[14]

The Cvek pulpotomy consists of (1) isolating the tooth with a dental dam, (2) disinfecting the tooth structure around the traumatic pulp exposure, (3) using a bur or diamond to gently remove pulp tissue to a depth of about 2 mm, (4) allowing bleeding to stop, (5) washing away the blood clot, (6) placing calcium hydroxide over the pulp wound, and finally (7) protecting the calcium hydroxide with a dental cement. The

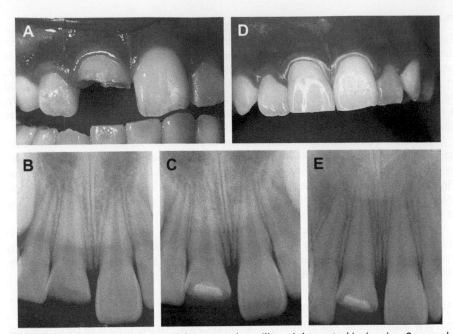

Fig. 4. Cvek pulpotomy technique. (*A*) Fractured maxillary right central incisor in a 9-year-old girl. The pulp was exposed. (*B*) Radiograph shows that the root is not fully developed. Note fairly wide-open apex. (*C*) Radiograph taken immediately after completion of the Cvek-type pulpotomy using calcium hydroxide as the capping agent. (*D*) Tooth restored with composite resin. (*E*) Radiograph taken 5 years after the pulpotomy procedure shows a mature, developed tooth. By comparing it to the adjacent left incisor, one can see that both teeth have developed similarly. (*Courtesy of* Leif K. Bakland, DDS, Loma Linda, CA.)

tooth can then be restored in a couple of ways: reattaching the broken fragment or restoring it with composite resin material.

Calcium hydroxide is initially an effective antibacterial material. However, calcium hydroxide loses its antibacterial capacity when it comes in contact with tissue fluid, which causes the calcium hydroxide to lose its high pH. Furthermore, calcium hydroxide is not a good material for sealing against bacterial penetration. So after the initial antibacterial stage, bacteria can readily penetrate any remaining calcium hydroxide. When using calcium hydroxide, it is therefore very important to cover the calcium hydroxide with a dental material that will resist bacterial penetration.

When using calcium hydroxide for pulp capping or pulpotomy, one depends on the material's ability to stimulate a hard-tissue bridge subjacent to the calcium hydroxide. After the initial hard tissue has formed across the pulpal wound, special cells form subjacent to the hard-tissue bridge. These cells become odontoblastlike cells and begin to form dentin after approximately 90 days. Provided the pulp remains healthy, this new dentin formation will continue at a normal pace, similar to formation in adjacent normal dentin areas (**Fig. 5**).[15]

The main problem with the use of calcium hydroxide is that one has to depend on the protection of the overlying dental filling material (eg, composite resin) to prevent bacterial penetration. By the time bacteria penetrate into the location of calcium hydroxide, the material has been neutralized by the adjacent tissue fluid. The necrotic zone generated initially by the calcium hydroxide's high pH now becomes an almost ideal incubation place for bacterial growth. When that happens, bacterial toxins can

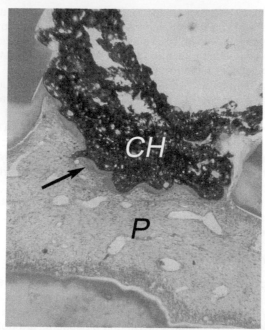

Fig. 5. Histologic picture (hematoxylin-eosin, magnification 156×) from an experiment on dogs' teeth showing the pulpal response to calcium hydroxide after 8 weeks. Note the newly developed hard tissue (*arrow*) between the calcium hydroxide (*CH*) and the pulp (*P*). (*From* Junn DJ. Quantitative assessment of dentin bridge formation following pulp capping with mineral trioxide aggregate. Master's thesis, Graduate School, Loma Linda University, 2000).

readily penetrate through the rather permeable hard-tissue bridge that formed in response to the calcium hydroxide and can cause serious pulpal damage.

One approach to the problem of bacterial invasion of the necrotic tissue between the newly formed hard-tissue bridge and the overlying dental restoration is to reenter the area, remove the necrotic remnants, and place a dental material (eg, composite resin) directly in contact with the newly formed bridge. It would be reasonable to consider performing such a procedure 6 to 12 months after the initial vital pulp therapy.[16]

Calcium hydroxide will continue to be an important material for vital pulp therapy. Its long record of usefulness means that calcium hydroxide can be used with predictability and its cost permits its ready access anywhere in the world.

A group of materials that have sparked much interest as potential materials for protection of exposed pulps are the resins. Much research has been conducted to find ways to use their ability to bond to tooth structure and thus protect the pulp from bacterial invasion. Successful application of resins has been mostly in the animal model while their use in humans has been less successful. While resins have a number of advocates promoting the use in pulp protection, there are also many who urge caution in their use.[17–20]

Recently, a new material, MTA, was developed. Initially made for sealing accidental root perforations occurring during endodontic procedures, MTA subsequently received considerable attention for its use in several other dental situations: as a root-end filling material, as an apical plug in roots with open apexes, and as a material for pulp capping and pulpotomy.[16]

The characteristics of MTA include biocompatibility and a close adaption to adjacent dentin, thus preventing bacterial leakage. Its pH is similar to that of calcium hydroxide so it may also have similar properties to calcium hydroxide. The fact that MTA is hydrophilic and needs moisture to cure makes it a most attractive material in many dental situations, including vital pulp therapy.[21]

It was shown in 1996 that MTA can be successfully used for pulpotomies.[22] The dentin forming subjacent to the MTA showed a normal configuration and formed faster than that forming under calcium hydroxide.[23] Because bacterial microleakage is a major concern with any dental material, it is noteworthy that MTA has been shown to resist bacterial penetration quite favorably compared to other materials.[24–26] Recently, Murray and colleagues[27] demonstrated that the pulp's reparative activity occurs more readily beneath capping materials that prevent bacterial microleakage, a feature favoring the use of MTA.

The major problem initially with the use of MTA for pulpotomies was that, because of its gray color, it tended to give the teeth a dark appearance. That problem has been corrected to a large extent by the development of a white MTA.[28]

VITAL PULP THERAPY TECHNIQUE

Vital pulp therapy can be performed on any tooth that has a vital, healthy pulp.[16] For practical reasons, it is primarily indicated for teeth in young patients in which continued root development is desirable. But the technique can also be used in the teeth of adults if extensive restorative/prosthetic procedures are not needed.

The technique for vital pulp therapy described here is that in which MTA is used (**Fig. 6**). However, the technique also applies to the use of calcium hydroxide; the main difference is that pulpal bleeding must be allowed to stop before calcium hydroxide can be placed on the wound while MTA can be placed in the presence of blood.

These are the recommended steps in performing vital pulp therapy for a tooth with traumatic pulp exposure:

1. Anesthetize, isolate with a dental dam, and disinfect the tooth and the fracture site.
   - The use of dental dam is important for minimizing bacterial contamination and for preventing chemicals and dental materials from spilling into the patient's mouth. Dentists interested in performing high-quality care will not confuse proper tooth isolation with the use of cotton rolls.
   - Disinfection of the fractured tooth can be done with sodium hypochlorite or with chlorhexidine. Both are excellent antiseptics and ensure a clean field.
2. Use a round diamond bur, or a straight diamond bur with a rounded tip, to gently cut into the pulp, starting at the exposure wound. The pulp removal should extend approximately 2 mm into the pulp proper. The cutting process must be done under a cooling water spray. The object is to create a 2-mm hole into the pulp tissue.
3. After the pulpotomy, allow initial bleeding to slow down. A small cotton pellet moistened with sodium hypochlorite can be used to help control the bleeding, wash away blood from the surrounding dentin, and ensure a disinfected field.
4. If calcium hydroxide is to be used for pulp protection, one must wait for bleeding to stop entirely, then gently wash away the blood clot and place the calcium hydroxide on the pulp wound followed by protective cement (eg, glass ionomer cement).
5. If MTA is to be used, it is not necessary to wait for the bleeding to stop completely. Mixed to manufacturer's recommendations (3:1, MTA/water), the prepared MTA has the consistency of wet sand. Excess moisture can be soaked up from the material with a cotton pellet. It is now ready to be placed in the pulpotomy cavity. It can be patted down into the cavity with a dry cotton pellet. It will take 3 to 4 hours to cure.

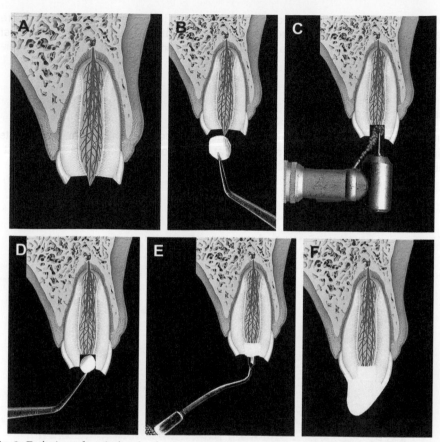

Fig. 6. Technique for vital pulp therapy using MTA. (*A*) Young, immature teeth with traumatic pulp exposure can be managed by protecting the pulp. (*B*) After anesthesia and isolation with a dental dam, the tooth is disinfected with either sodium hypochlorite or chlorhexidine. (*C*) A shallow pulpotomy into the stroma of the pulp is made with a high-speed bur or diamond instrument. (*D*) Control of bleeding and disinfection can be accomplished using a cotton pellet moistened with sodium hypochlorite. (*E*) MTA is gently placed into the pulpotomy site, covering the pulp wound. (*F*) The tooth can be restored after the MTA has cured (usually within 3–4 hours) or immediately by protecting the MTA first with a glass ionomer cement. (*From* Andreasen JO, Andresen FM, Bakland LK, et al. Traumatic dental injuries. A manual. 2nd edition. Oxford [United Kingdom]: Blackwell Munksgaard; 2003. p. 59; with permission.)

A question that comes up with respect to the use of MTA for vital pulp therapy is: Does it need to be protected during the curing process?

Before it cures to its solid state, MTA can easily be washed away if subjected to extensive flow of any fluid. However, if it is only exposed to a moist environment, such as in the mouth, and the patient refrains from drinking and eating for 3 to 4 hours, the material will cure satisfactorily. In fact, the moisture in the mouth will help in curing the material.

The options for the management of the tooth immediately after the MTA pulpotomy are to (1) allow the MTA to cure in contact with saliva in the mouth, (2) protect the tooth with a temporary crown, or (3) proceed with the restoration of the tooth immediately because moisture for curing will come from the fluid in the subjacent pulp tissue. There are not sufficient data available to determine which of these methods will give the best outcome. It is likely that the care used in performing any treatment is the most important predictor of outcome.

TREATMENT OUTCOME

Clinical reports indicate that the MTA pulpotomy procedure can provide good results (**Fig. 7**).[29–31] Such good results stem from at least two factors: favorable biocompatibility and sealing ability of MTA.

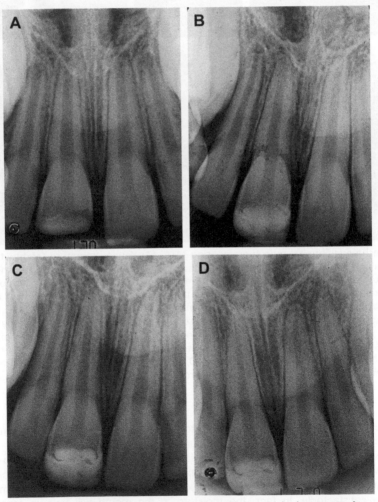

Fig. 7. Pulpotomy using MTA. (*A*) Radiograph of a complicated (pulp exposure) crown fracture of the maxillary right central incisor. Note immature root development. (*B*) Radiograph taken immediately after vital pulp therapy. (*C*) Radiograph taken 1 year postoperatively. (*D*) Radiograph taken 4 years postoperatively. Note the appearance of normal root development when compared to the adjacent incisor. (*Courtesy of* John Pratte, La Canada, CA.)

Early in the development of MTA, it was tested for biocompatibility and responded most favorably.[28,32,33] This is important for a clinical situation, such as providing a favorable environment for new hard-tissue (dentin) formation. Studies have shown that dentin formation under MTA is of very good quality.[21–23]

Bacterial leakage is a big problem with all dental materials. Some, such as gutta-percha, allow considerable leakage, while others—and MTA belongs to this group— are quite resistant to bacterial penetration. Several studies have demonstrated that MTA is one of the best materials with respect to preventing leakage of all kinds.[24–26]

In contrast to calcium hydroxide, which creates a zone of necrosis when it comes in contact with vital tissues, such as the pulp, MTA appears to stimulate hard-tissue formation without at first causing any tissue damage.[21,23,27,31,32] The zone of necrosis below calcium hydroxide does initiate a hard-tissue bridge, but if subsequently there is bacterial leakage around the crown restoration, the bacteria can colonize the zone of necrosis, resulting in pulpal damage from bacterial toxins that can penetrate the permeable hard-tissue bridge. Therefore, when using calcium hydroxide for vital pulp therapy in teeth with crown fractures, as mentioned above, one should consider placing a new filling after the formation of a hard-tissue bridge.

Because MTA does not produce a zone of necrosis and because it provides good protection against bacterial leakage, it is not necessary to replace the MTA once the new dentin has formed subjacent to the material.

Animal research and case reports have indicated that MTA is a suitable material for vital pulp therapy.[21–23,29–31] In its early formulation, the gray color was a problem when the material was used in the crown of a tooth. This has been improved with the intro-duction a few years ago of white MTA. There may still be instances of a slight discol-oration even with the white material, but that may be managed by veneering the crown if necessary.

The importance of preventing the loss of teeth, particularly anterior teeth, in young patients cannot be overstated. Crown fractures, if managed properly, need not result in loss of such teeth or, in most cases, the loss of pulps. Preserving pulp vitality ensures maturation of the roots, which prevents cervical root fractures frequently seen in young teeth with premature loss of vital pulps.

REFERENCES

1. Herman BW. Biologische Wurzelbehandlung. Frankfurt am Main: W. Kramer & Co; 1936.
2. Zander FJ. Reaction of the pulp to calcium hydroxide. J Dent Res 1939;6:373–9.
3. Bogen G, Kim JS, Bakland LK. Direct pulp capping with mineral trioxide aggre-gate. An observational study. J Am Dent Assoc 2008;139:305–15.
4. Andreasen JO, Andreasen FM, Bakland LK, et al. Traumatic dental injuries. A manual. edition 2. Oxford, UK: Blackwell Munkgaard; 2003.
5. Robertson A, Andreasen FM, Andreasen JO, et al. Long-term prognosis of crown-fractured permanent incisors. The effect of stage of root development and asso-ciated luxation injury. Int J Paediatr Dent 2000;10:191–9.
6. Cvek M. Partial pulpotomy in crown fractured incisors: results 3 to 15 years after treatment. Acta Stomatol Croat 1993;27:167–73.
7. Heide S. The effect of pulp capping and pulpotomy on hard tissue bridges of contaminated pulps. Int Endod J 1991;24:126–34.
8. Fuks AB, Chosack A, Klein H, et al. Partial pulpotomy as a treatment alternative for exposed pulps in crown fractured permanent incisors. Endod Dent Traumatol 1987;3:100–2.

9. Lam RV. Contour changes of the alveolar process following extractions. J Prosthet Dent 1960;10:25–32.
10. Farik B, Kreiborg S, Andreasen JO. Adhesive bonding of fragmented anterior teeth. Endod Dent Traumatol 1998;14:119–23.
11. DiAngelis AJ. Bonding of fractured tooth segments: a review of the past 20 years. J Calif Dent Assoc J 1998;26:753–9.
12. Bakland LK, Andreasen JO. Dental traumatology: essential diagnosis and treatment planning. Endod Topics 2004;7:14–34.
13. Cox CF, Keall CL, Keall HJ, et al. Biocompatibility of surface-sealed dental materials against exposed pulps. J Prosthet Dent 1987;57:1–8.
14. Cvek M. A clinical report on partial pulpotomy and capping with calcium hydroxide in permanent incisors with complicated crown fractures. J Endod 1978;4:232–7.
15. Schröder U. The effect of calcium hydroxide–containing pulp capping agents on pulp cell migration, proliferation, and cell differentiation. J Dent Res 1985;64:541–8.
16. Bakland LK. New endodontic procedures using mineral trioxide aggregate (MTA) for teeth with traumatic injuries. In: Andreasen JO, Andreasen FM, Andersson L, editors. Textbook and color atlas of traumatic injuries to the teeth. 4th edition. Oxford: Blackwell Munksgaard; 2006.
17. Schuurs AHB, Gruythuysen RJM, Wesselink PR. Pulp capping with adhesive resin-based composite vs. calcium hydroxide: a review. Endod Dent Traumatol 2000;16:240–50.
18. Olsburgh S, Jacoby T, Krejci I. Crown fractures in the permanent dentition: pulpal and restorative considerations. Dent Traumatol 2002;18:103–15.
19. Costa CAS, Oliveira MF, Giro EMA, et al. Biocompatibility of resin-based materials used as pulp-capping agents. Int Endod J 2003;36:831–9.
20. Hörsted-Bindslev P, Vilkinis V, Sidlauskas A. Direct capping of human pulps with dentin bonding system or calcium hydroxide cement. Oral Surg Oral Med Oral Pathol Oral Radiol Endod 2003;96:591–600.
21. Pitt Ford TR, Torabinejad M, Abedi HR, et al. Using mineral trioxide aggregate as a pulp-capping material. J Am Dent Assoc 1996;127:1491–4.
22. Abedi HR, Torabinejad M, Pitt Ford TR, et al. The use of mineral trioxide aggregate cement (MTA) as a direct pulp capping agent. J Endod 1996;22:199. [Abstract #44].
23. Junn DJ. Quantitative assessment of dentin bridge formation following pulp capping with mineral trioxide aggregate. Master's thesis, Graduate School, Loma Linda University, 2000.
24. Lee SJ, Monsef M, Torabinejad M. The sealing ability of a mineral trioxide aggregate for repair of lateral root perforations. J Endod 1993;19:541–4.
25. Torabinejad M, Rastegar AF, Kettering JD, et al. Bacterial leakage of mineral trioxide aggregate as a root end filling material. J Endod 1995;21:109–21.
26. Bates CF, Carnes DL, del Rio CE. Longitudinal sealing ability of mineral trioxide aggregate as a root-end filling material. J Endod 1996;22:575–8.
27. Murray PE, Hafez AA, Smith AJ, et al. Histomorphometric analysis of odontoblast-like cell numbers and dentin bridge secretory activity following pulp exposure. Int Endod J 2003;36:106–16.
28. Camilleri J, Montesin FE, Papaioannou S, et al. Biocompatibility of two commercial forms of mineral trioxide aggregate. Int Endod J 2004;37:699–704.
29. Aeinenchi M, Eslami B, Ghanbariha M, et al. Mineral trioxide aggregate (MTA) and calcium hydroxide as pulp-capping agents in human teeth: a preliminary report. Int Endod J 2002;36:225–31.

30. Witherspoon DE, Small JC, Harris GZ. Mineral trioxide aggregate pulpotomies: a case series outcomes assessment. J Am Dent Assoc 2006;137:610–8.
31. Iwamoto CE, Adachi E, Pameijer CH, et al. Clinical and histological evaluation of white MTA in direct pulp capping. Am J Dent 2006;19:85–90.
32. Koh ET, McDonald R, Pitt Ford TR, et al. Cellular response to mineral trioxide aggregate. J Endod 1998;24:543–7.
33. Mitchell PJ, Pitt Ford TR, Torabinejad M, et al. Osteoblast biocompatibility of mineral trioxide aggregate. Biomaterials 1999;20:167–73.

Management of Trauma to Supporting Dental Structures

Husam Elias, MD, DMD[a],*, Dale A. Baur, DDS, MD[b]

KEYWORDS

- Trauma • Teeth • Mandible • Maxilla • Alveolar process
- Fracture • Management

Teeth, periodontium, and supporting alveolar bone are frequently involved in trauma and account for approximately 15% of all emergency room visits. The cause of the dentoalveolar trauma varies in different demographics but generally results from falls, playground accidents, domestic violence, bicycle accidents, motor vehicle accidents, assaults, altercations, and sports injuries. Gassner and colleagues[1] reported an incidence of 48.25% in all facial injuries, 57.8% in play and household accidents, 50.1% in sports accidents, 38.6% in accidents at work, 35.8% in acts of violence, 34.2% in traffic accidents, and 31% in unspecified accidents. Falling is the primary cause of dentoalveolar trauma in early childhood. Andreasen[2] reported a bimodal trend in the peak incidence of dentoalveolar trauma in children aged 2 to 4 and 8 to 10 years. Likewise, there is an overall prevalence of 11% to 30% in children with primary dentition, and 5% to 20% in permanent and mixed dentition, with a ratio of 2:1 male to female. Of dental trauma repoted, falls accounted for 49%, sports-related injuries accounted for 18%, bicycle and scooter accidents accounted for 13%, assault accounted for 7%, and road traffic accidents accounted for 1.5% of all injuries.[3]

Predisposing factors include abnormal occlusions, overjet exceeding 4 mm, labially inclined incisors, lip incompetence, a short upper lip, and mouth breathing.[4] These conditions can be seen in individuals with class II division I malocclusions or oral habits such as thumb sucking. A significant number of dentoalveolar injuries are associated with the management of the comatose patient[5] or the patient undergoing general anesthesia. Lockhart and colleagues[6] surveyed 133 directors of training programs in anesthesiology and found that on average of 1 in every 1000 tracheal intubations resulted in dental trauma. They also reported that 90% of the dental complications may have been prevented with a screening dental examination of the patient and the use of mouth protectors.[7]

[a] Head & Neck Institute, Cleveland Clinic, Room A/70, 9500 Euclid Avenue, Cleveland, OH 44195, USA
[b] Department of Oral and Maxillofacial Surgery, Case Western Reserve University, 2123 Abington Road, Cleveland, OH 44106–4905, USA
* Corresponding author.
E-mail address: dale.baur@case.edu (H. Elias).

Dent Clin N Am 53 (2009) 675–689
doi:10.1016/j.cden.2009.08.003
0011-8532/09/$ – see front matter

dental.theclinics.com

PATIENT EVALUATION

Dentoalveolar injuries should be considered an emergency situation because successful management of the injury requires proper diagnosis and treatment within a limited time to achieve more favorable outcomes. The initial evaluation must include a general assessment of the patient's overall condition—not only past medical history but also time, place, and mechanism of trauma and associated injuries. Immediate pain relief and reduction of dental and alveolar injuries allow for better assessment of the dentition.

HISTORY

The history obtained from patients with dentoalveolar injury should include the following information:

1. Biographic and demographic data, including name, age, gender, and race.
2. The time interval between the injury and presentation to the clinic or emergency department. The success of managing luxated teeth, crown fractures, and alveolar bone fractures may be influenced by delayed treatment.
3. The site of the accident, which may provide clues to the degree of bacterial contamination and possible need for tetanus prophylaxis.
4. The nature of the accident, which can provide insight into the type of injury to be suspected. For example, a fall often causes injury to the maxillary anterior dentition, but a blow to the chin frequently causes crown-root fractures of the premolars or molars along with symphyseal or condylar fractures of the mandible. In children and women, if the history of the injury does not correspond to the type of injury expected, abuse should be considered. The clinician should carefully document the findings and discussion with the patient. The nature of the injury also may provide information regarding other associated occult injuries. For example, an occult injury to the neck should be ruled out during the examination of the patient who has been thrown forward against the dashboard as an unrestrained passenger or against the guardrail from a bicycle accident.
5. Information related to the events surrounding the accident, including whether teeth or pieces of teeth were noted at the accident site. Unless all crowns and teeth are accounted for, radiographic examination of the periapical tissues, chest, abdominal region, and the perioral soft tissue should be performed to ascertain whether the missing fragments of teeth are in these tissues or body cavities. The clinician should determine whether the patient or parent replanted any partially or completely avulsed teeth and how a tooth was stored before presentation to the dentist or the emergency room. Finally, information should be obtained about whether the patient had loss of consciousness, confusion, nausea, vomiting, or visual disturbances after the accident. If any of these symptoms occurred, intracranial injury should be suspected and the patient should be referred for immediate neurologic evaluation. Treatment of the dentoalveolar injury can be delayed until such evaluation is completed.
6. Changes in the occlusion as a result of the injury, which could indicate tooth displacement or dentoalveolar and/or jaw fractures.
7. Medical and dental history, which may delay or modify treatments, including the presence of major systemic illness such as bleeding disorders or epilepsy.

CLINICAL EXAMINATION

An important aspect of the physical examination is the overall evaluation of the physical status of the patient. Guided by the findings of the history, the patient should be examined for the presence of concomitant injury, including measurement of vital signs such as pulse rate, blood pressure, and respiration. Significant changes may indicate intracranial injury, cervical spine injury, chest or abdominal injury, or even aspiration of an avulsed tooth. The patient's mental status also should be assessed by asking specific questions and observing the patient's reaction and behavior during the history and examinations. Once a general examination is completed and any concomitant injury is ruled out, the oral and maxillofacial examination is performed.

1. Extraoral soft tissue examinations include inspection of the soft tissue for lacerations, abrasions, and contusions of the skin of the face, chin, forehead, and scalp. The depth, location, and proximity to vital structures of any lacerations should be noted, recorded, and considered when the lacerations are repaired. Location of laceration may suggest the site of dental injury. The temporomandibular joint is palpated and range of jaw motion determined to rule out condylar fracture.

2. Intraoral soft tissue examination includes assessment for injuries of the oral mucosa and gingiva and laceration of the lips, tongue, floor of the mouth, and cheek. Such injuries require thorough evaluation for the presence of foreign bodies, debris, and teeth or teeth fragments embedded within the tissue. It may be necessary to clean the laceration and the oral cavity to remove any clots and stop active bleeding to conduct an adequate examination. Gingival lacerations are often indications of tooth displacement, and bleeding from nonlacerated marginal gingival frequently is indicative of periodontal ligament damage or mandibular fracture. It is important to account for all teeth; missing teeth or pieces of teeth that have not been left at the scene of the accident should be considered to have been aspirated, swallowed, or displaced into the soft tissues, nasal cavity, or maxillary sinus until proven otherwise. These areas should be examined radiographically to rule out the presence of teeth or fragments.

3. Examination of the jaws and alveolar bone. Fractures of the alveolar process are readily detected by visual inspection and often manifested as gingival laceration. In the absence of such laceration, manual palpation of fractured segments of the alveolar process usually reveals mobility and crepitation of the fragments. Fractures of the underlying bone can be detected by the presence of gross malocclusion, pain, and mobility of the fractured segment to palpation. Bleeding from the gingival crevice of a tooth, vertical laceration of the attached mucosa, and submucosal ecchymosis of the floor of the mouth are other signs of jaw fracture.

4. Before examining the teeth for fractures, they should be cleansed of blood and debris. Any infraction (cracks through the enamel) or fractures of the crowns should be noted. Infraction lines can be detected by directing a light beam parallel to the long axis of the tooth. Crown fractures should be evaluated to determine extension into the dentin and the pulp. The size and location of pulp exposures, if present, should be recorded. Crown-root fractures in all quadrants also should be evaluated. Changes in the color of traumatized teeth and translucency may indicate exposed pulp. It is important to remember that indirect trauma leading to crown-root fractures in one quadrant is often accompanied by similar fractures of the same side of the opposing jaw. Displacement of teeth from dentoalveolar trauma usually can be detected by visual examination. Examination of the occlusion may help to detect minor degrees of tooth movements. Although teeth may be displaced in any direction, the most common displacement is buccolingually. The direction and extent of displacement should be recorded. Lateral luxation and intrusion of teeth may cause minimal clinical symptoms because the teeth remain located in this displaced position. Lingual displacement of the apex of primary teeth

can interfere with permanent successors. All teeth should be tested for horizontal and axial mobility. If a tooth does not appear to be displaced but is mobile, a root fracture should be suspected. In such instances, the location of the fracture usually determines the degree of mobility. Movement of the tooth being tested, together with the adjacent tooth, suggests dentoalveolar fracture. The purpose of vitality testing is to register the conduction of stimuli to the sensory receptors of the dental pulp. This test can be performed using mechanical stimulation with cotton soaked in saline or by thermal test using treated guttapercha, ice, ethyl chloride, carbon dioxide snow, dichloro-difluormethane, or electric vitalometers. The test may be difficult to perform or be relatively unreliable in the acute setting after traumatic injury, however. Results also can be unreliable in uncooperative children. Results may be more accurate when pulp testing is performed several weeks later; such tests should be performed before endodontic therapy.

RADIOGRAPHIC EVALUATION

Indications for radiographic examinations are as follows:

1. Presence of root fractures
2. Degree of extrusion or intrusion
3. Presence of pre-existing periodontal disease
4. Extent of root development
5. Size of the pulp chamber
6. Presence of jaw fractures
7. Tooth fragments and foreign bodies lodged in soft tissues

Radiographic examination is essential to determine whether any underlying structures are damaged and should include periapical, occlusal, and panoramic radiographs. The periapical radiograph provides the most detailed information about root fractures and the dislocation of teeth. After treatment, periapical films can confirm the proper positioning of an avulsed or luxated tooth into the alveolus. Occlusal radiographs, however, provide a larger field of view, and the detail is almost as sharp as a periapical radiograph.

When occlusal radiographs or periapical films are used to examine soft tissues for the presence of foreign bodies, reduce the radiographic exposure time. The panoramic radiograph is a useful screening view and can demonstrate fractures of the mandible and maxilla and fractures of the alveolar ridges and teeth. In the hospital setting, dental radiographs may not be available. Although not ideal, plain films, such as the mandibular series and the Caldwell views, may reveal tooth and alveolar injuries. In the trauma patient whose tooth has not been accounted for at the accident scene, arrange for chest films to rule out the possibility of aspiration. Abdominal radiographic films can determine whether displaced teeth or prosthetic appliances have been ingested.

CLASSIFICATION
Injuries to the Periodontal Tissues

Concussion
A concussion is an injury to the tooth-supporting structures without abnormal loosening or displacement of the tooth but with marked reaction to percussion.

Subluxation (loosening)
Subluxation is an injury to the tooth-supporting structures with abnormal loosening but without displacement of the tooth.

Intrusive luxation (central dislocation)
Intrusive luxation (**Fig. 1**) is displacement of the tooth into the alveolar bone with comminution or fracture of the alveolar socket.

Extrusive luxation (peripheral dislocation, partial avulsion)
An extrusive luxation is partial displacement of the tooth out of the alveolar socket.

Lateral luxation
A lateral luxation is displacement of the tooth in a direction other than axially, accompanied by a comminution or fracture of the alveolar socket.

Retained root fracture
A retained root fracture (**Fig. 2**) is a fracture with retention of the root segment but loss of the crown segment out of the socket.

Exarticulation (complete avulsion)
An exarticulation is a complete displacement of a tooth out of the alveolar socket.

Injuries to the Supporting Bone

Comminution of the alveolar socket
Crushing and comminution of the alveolar socket (**Fig. 3**) can occur together with intrusive and lateral luxation.

Fracture of the alveolar socket wall
A fracture of the alveolar socket is confined to the facial or lingual socket wall.

Fracture of the alveolar process
A fracture of the alveolar process (**Fig. 4**) may or may not involve the alveolar socket.

Fractures of the mandible or maxilla
A fracture involving the base of the mandible or maxilla (**Fig. 5**)—and often the alveolar process—may or may not involve the alveolar socket.

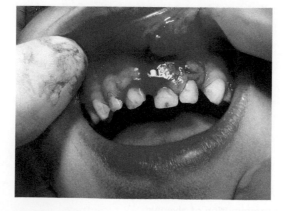

Fig. 1. Luxation.

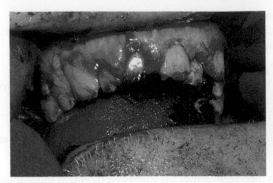

Fig. 2. Retained root fractures.

Injuries to the Gingiva or Oral Mucosa

Laceration of gingiva or oral mucosa
A shallow or deep wound in the mucosa results from a tear and is usually produced by a sharp object.

Contusion of gingiva or mucosa
A bruise is usually produced by impact from a blunt object and results in submucosal hemorrhage without a break in the mucosa.

Abrasion of gingiva or oral mucosa
A superficial wound produced by rubbing or scraping of the mucosa, which leaves a raw, bleeding surface, constitutes an abrasion of the gingiva or oral mucosa.

MANAGEMENT
General Considerations

The overall goal of treatment is to preserve the functional state of teeth, bone, and gingiva. Although every attempt should be made to maintain all of these structures permanently, it may be necessary either to sacrifice or only temporarily maintain teeth. The final restorative plan should be taken into consideration when deciding whether and when to remove teeth or bony segments at the initial phase of treatment. The periodontal status of the teeth in the alveolar fracture should be assessed, and attempts to maintain teeth that would be otherwise unsalvageable for periodontal reasons should be avoided. Teeth that would not be useful in the final restorative plan and are

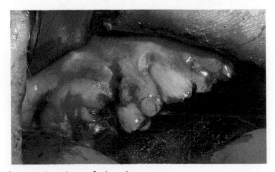

Fig. 3. Crushing and comminution of alveolus.

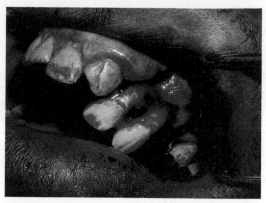

Fig. 4. Fracture of alveolar process.

condemned are sometimes retained temporarily in alveolar fractures to preserve the bone that would otherwise have to be removed when removing the teeth. Preserving the bone maintains proper alveolar contour and bulk, which often results in more satisfactory dental rehabilitation.

Management of Injuries to the Periodontal Tissues

Luxation injuries occur in the permanent and primary dentition. Etiologic factors in the permanent dentition include bicycle accidents, sports injuries, falls, and fights, whereas falls dominate in the primary dentition. In both types of dentition, luxation is most commonly seen in the maxillary central incisor region. The type of luxation injury depends on the type of force and the direction of impact. In the primary dentition, intrusions and extrusions make up most of all injuries,[8] probably because of the resilient nature of the alveolar bone in children of this age, whereas intrusion injuries are markedly reduced in the permanent dentition. More frequently, 2 or more teeth are luxated simultaneously, and concomitant crown or root fractures occur. Diagnosis of the type of luxation injury depends wholly on clinical and radiographic examination. Common sequelae of intrusion injuries are pulp canal obliteration, pulp necrosis, internal resorption, external resorption, marginal bone loss, and transient apical breakdown, each of which depends on the type of injury, maturity of the affected tooth, and subsequent treatment intervention.[9,10]

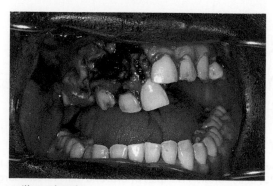

Fig. 5. Fracture of maxillary alveolus.

Management of Injuries to the Supporting Bone

Fractures of the alveolar process

These injuries can be associated with dental luxation injuries, maxillar or mandibular fractures, or isolated. Alveolar fractures are managed by immediate closed reduction of the fracture to realign the segments, reduce the teeth, and align them and place in occlusion. Splinting with a rigid splint using acid-etched resin or orthodontic brackets and wire on either side of the fractured alveolus for 4 to 6 weeks is an option. If the fracture involves only the alveolar segment and there is no associated luxation injury, then closed reduction and fixation is performed with a single arch bar and 24- or 26-gauge wire for 4 weeks. Rigid fixation can be applied using mini or micro titanium plates and screws to fixate the fractures, with special attention paid to placing teeth in the correct occlusion during fixation.[11–14]

Fractures of the maxilla and mandible

The maxilla can be fractured at different levels based on the level of injury (**Fig. 6**). Le Fort I fractures (horizontal fractures) may result from a force of injury directed low on the maxillary alveolar rim in a downward direction. This fracture is also known as a Guerin fracture or "floating palate" and usually involves the inferior nasal aperture. The fracture extends from the nasal septum to the lateral pyriform rims, travels horizontally above the teeth apices, crosses below the zygomaticomaxillary junction, and traverses the pterygomaxillary junction to interrupt the pterygoid plates.

Le Fort II fractures (pyramidal fractures) may result from a blow to the lower or mid maxilla and usually involve the inferior orbital rim. Such a fracture has a pyramidal shape and extends from the nasal bridge at or below the nasofrontal suture through the frontal processes of the maxilla, inferolaterally through the lacrimal bones and inferior orbital floor and rim through or near the inferior orbital foramen, and inferiorly through the anterior wall of the maxillary sinus. It then travels under the zygoma, across the pterygomaxillary fissure, and through the pterygoid plates.

Le Fort III fractures (transverse fractures) are otherwise known as craniofacial dissociation and involve the zygomatic arch. They may follow impact to the nasal bridge or upper maxilla. These fractures start at the nasofrontal and frontomaxillary sutures and extend posteriorly along the medial wall of the orbit through the nasolacrimal groove

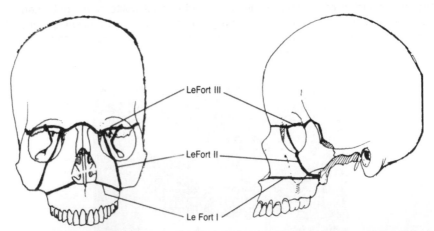

Fig. 6. Diagram showing various levels of Le Fort fractures. (*Adapted from* Peterson LJ, Indresano AT, Marciani RD, et al, editors. Principles of oral and maxillofacial surgery. Philadelphia: Lippincott-Raven; 1992. p. 471; with permission.)

and ethmoid bones. The thicker sphenoid bone posteriorly usually prevents continuation of the fracture into the optic canal. Instead, the fracture continues along the floor of the orbit along the inferior orbital fissure and continues superolaterally through the lateral orbital wall, through the zygomaticofrontal junction and the zygomatic arch. Intranasally, a branch of the fracture extends through the base of the perpendicular plate of the ethmoid, through the vomer, and through the interface of the pterygoid plates to the base of the sphenoid.

Le Fort I fractures affect the dentoalveolar complex most frequently and are often combined with alveolar process fractures or luxation injuries. These fractures are managed based on their severity. Maxillomandibular fixation is used to re-establish the occlusion as the first step followed by exposure of the fractures via a circumvestibular incision (**Fig. 7**), and fixation of bony segments can be achieved with mini or micro plates and screws.[13]

The mandible can injured in at several different sites, namely the body of the mandible, which is the molar-premolar area, symphysis in the midline, parasymphysis at the canine-premolar area, the angle area (**Fig. 8**), and condyles. Mandible fractures are classified as favorable or unfavorable, depending on the orientation of the fracture and associated muscle pull. Unfavorable fractures are a result of muscle pull, which causes the segments to separate. On the other hand, fractures are favorable when muscle pull results in reduction of the fractured segments (**Figs. 9** and **10**). Fractures also can be classified as compound, greenstick, comminuted, telescoped, direct, indirect, and pathologic.

The diagnosis of the mandibular fracture is typically based on clinical findings, whereas imaging studies are used to confirm the diagnosis. Patients present with complaints of pain, mal-occlusion, inability to chew, and difficulty opening. Frequently these patients present with paresthesia of the mental nerve on the fractured side. On physical examination, there is associated edema, a hematoma of the floor of the mouth (**Fig. 11**), and lacerations of the gingiva or skin adjacent to the fracture site. The clinician needs to be aware that up to 60% of mandibular fractures are bilateral in nature because of the unique shape of the mandible. Common fracture combinations include the angle area on one side and the opposite parasymphysis, bilateral parasymphysis areas, angle and opposite condyles, bilateral angle fractures, or bilateral condyle fractures, which can occur with a direct blow to the chin. The most useful imaging for diagnosis and management of mandible fractures is a panoramic radiograph in conjunction with a CT scan. The most common site for a mandibular fracture to occur is the body area (**Fig. 12**).

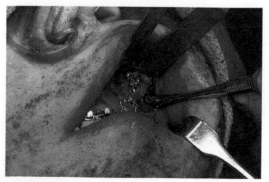

Fig. 7. Open reduction with internal fixation of Le Fort fracture with plate and screws.

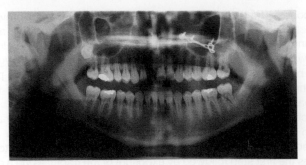

Fig. 8. Mandibular fracture through left second molar. The second molar would need to be extracted. Note hardware on left maxilla from previous surgery.

Questions frequently arise regarding the management of teeth in the line of fracture. Generally speaking, a tooth in the line of fracture should be removed if it excessively mobile, periodontally involved, or nonrestorable, if more than 50% of the root surface is exposed in the fracture line, or if the tooth prevents proper reduction of the fracture. Teeth should be retained if they are otherwise healthy and contribute to fracture reduction and stabilization.

Antibiotic coverage is indicated in mandibular fractures, especially with fractures in the tooth-bearing segments of the mandible, because there is direct contact with the oral environment and a high incidence of infection. With modern low-profile titanium hardware currently available, mandibular fractures are often treated with open reduction and internal fixation (ORIF). Access is gained to the mandible through transoral or skin incisions. The advantage of ORIF includes immediate mobilization of the mandible, although the patient needs to maintain a nonchewing diet for 4 to 6 weeks. With the use of ORIF, bony fractures heal by primary intention because the fracture is anatomically reduced (**Fig. 13**). Disadvantages of ORIF include increased operating room time and the occasional need for skin incisions.

A still reliable technique for managing mandible fractures is maxillomandibular fixation (MMF). Erich arch bars or MMF screws are used to immobilize the fracture (**Fig. 14**). The disadvantage of this technique is that 4 to 6 weeks of immobilization is necessary for satisfactory healing. Bony healing occurs by secondary intention with the formation of a healing callus. Advantages of this technique include rapid

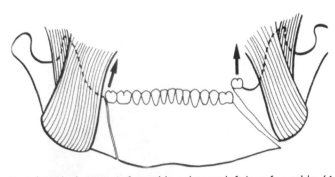

Fig. 9. Patient's right side fracture is favorable, whereas left is unfavorable. (*Adapted from* Peterson LJ, Indresano AT, Marciani RD, et al, editors. Principles of oral and maxillofacial surgery. Philadelphia: Lippincott-Raven; 1992. p. 410; with permission.)

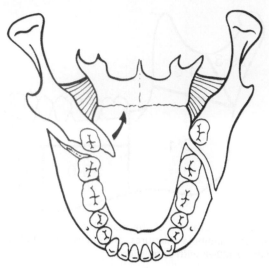

Fig. 10. Patient's left side fracture is favorable, whereas right is unfavorable. (*Adapted from* Peterson LJ, Indresano AT, Marciani RD, et al, editors. Principles of oral and maxillofacial surgery. Philadelphia: Lippincott-Raven; 1992. p. 411; with permission.)

treatment time, and general anesthesia is not always required. MMF is not indicated in patients who may be unable to tolerate prolonged periods of immobilization (eg, patients with seizure disorders, chronic alcoholics, and some psychiatric patients).

Condylar fractures present a unique subset of mandibular fractures. Patients present with complaints of malocclusion and pain in the condylar area. On physical examination, these patients have decreased range of motion, may have blood in the external auditory canal, and deviate on opening to the fractured side. There is frequently premature occlusion on the fractured side with a contralateral posterior open bite. In cases of bilateral condylar fractures, there is usually an anterior open bite. Imaging should include a panoramic radiograph and a CT scan.

The management of condylar fractures remains a somewhat controversial issue. For adults, management options include an open surgical approach versus closed reduction with MMF. Absolute indications for open surgical management of a fractured

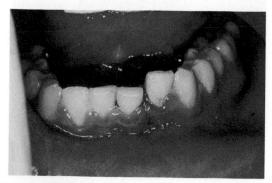

Fig. 11. Mandible fracture. Note floor of mouth hematoma and occlusal step.

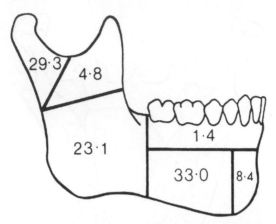

Fig. 12. Incidence of fracture locations of the mandible. (*Adapted from* Ellis E, Moos KF, El-Attar A. Ten years of mandibular fractures: an analysis of 2,137 cases. Oral Surg Oral Med Oral Pathol 1985;59:120–9; with permission.)

condyle are lateral dislocation of the condylar head, fracture into the middle cranial fossa, a foreign body within the joint, or when the condylar segment prevents manipulation of the mandible into the proper occlusion. Relative indications for a surgical management include cases with bilateral condylar fractures and associated mid-face fractures. In these cases, it is necessary to establish the proper vertical and horizontal position of the mandible, which then allows for proper reduction of the mid-face fractures. Another relative indication for open reduction of a condylar fracture includes situations in which patients are unwilling or unable to tolerate MMF. The surgical approach to a fractured condyle is through a preauricular skin incision, with careful dissection and preservation of the facial nerve.

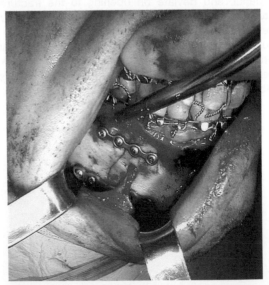

Fig. 13. Note close anatomic reduction of fracture with ORIF. Mental nerve is visualized and intact.

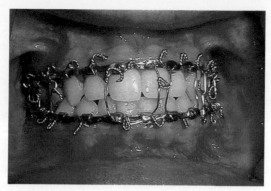

Fig. 14. Arch bars in position with good occlusal relationship.

MMF is frequently used to manage condylar fractures instead of surgery. If MMF is applied, the length of immobilization is shorter than for other mandible fractures because the risk of ankylosis is greater when the condyle is involved. For this reason, patients are kept in wire fixation for 7 to 10 days only. At that time, orthodontic elastics are used to allow for some mobility but simultaneously maintain the pretrauma dental occlusion. In children with condylar fractures, the risk of ankylosis is high because of the rapid healing potential of their bone (**Fig. 15**). MMF, if used, should only be applied for 5 to 7 days. At that time, physical therapy is initiated to prevent ankylosis and regain mandibular range of motion. If necessary, light guiding orthodontic elastics can be used to help maintain the appropriate occlusal relationships. Most surgeons avoid open management of condylar fractures in children to avoid disturbing the condylar growth center.[13]

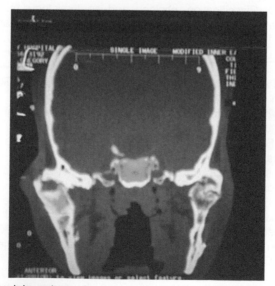

Fig. 15. CT scan of adult patient who sustained bilateral condylar fractures as a child. He subsequently developed bilateral TMJ ankylosis.

Management of Injuries to the Gingival and Oral Mucosa

The goal in management of injuries to soft tissue is to maintain vascularity of the soft tissue to aid in healing of the underlying bone and prevent devitalization and optimize gingival healing to prevent future recession and root exposure.

Contusion

Bleeding in the subcutaneous tissue without surface epithelial break results in ecchymosis and possible hematoma. These injuries are usually self-limiting and do not require special care. Antibiotic coverage is seldom necessary.

Abrasion

These are superficial injuries wherein epithelial tissues are worn, scratched, or rubbed. Treatment includes local cleansing, especially removal of foreign bodies imbedded in the abrasion to prevent tattooing. Antibiotic coverage is seldom necessary.

Laceration

Laceration is the most common form of injury. Gingival and mucosal laceration should be repaired to decrease the risk of bone and root exposure after careful inspection and cleansing of the lacerations for any foreign bodies. Devitalized tissues should be excised conservatively, especially at the keratinized gingival level. Gingiva should be reapproximated using resorbable or nonresorbable sutures sized as 4–0 or 5–0. Mucosa should be reapproximated in similar manner. Perioral muscles are occasionally lacerated and need to be reattached carefully. Sliding and advancement flaps may be required to cover bone and root in cases of tissue avulsion.

REFERENCES

1. Gassner R, Bösch R, Tuli T, et al. Prevalence of dental trauma in 6000 patients with facial injuries: implications for prevention. Oral Surg Oral Med Oral Pathol Oral Radiol Endod 1999;87(1):27–33.
2. Andreasen JO. Classification, etiology and epidemiology. In: Andreasen JO, editor. Traumatic injuries of the teeth. 2nd edition. Copenhagen (Denmark): Munksgaard; 1981. p. 19.
3. Lephart SM, Fu FH. Emergency treatment of athletic injuries. Dent Clin North Am 1991;35:707.
4. Wright G, Bell A, McGlashan G, et al. Dentoalveolar trauma in Glasgow: an audit of mechanism and injury. Dent Traumatol 2007;23(4):226–31.
5. Piercell MP, White DE, Nelson R. Prevention of self-inflicted trauma in semicomatose patients. J Oral Surg 1974;32:903.
6. Lockhart PB, Feldbau EV, Gabel RA, et al. Dental complications during and after tracheal intubation. J Am Dent Assoc 1986;112:480.
7. Aromaa U, Pesonen P, Linko K, et al. Difficulties with tooth protectors in endotracheal intubation. Acta Anaesthesiol Scand 1988;32:304.
8. FitzGerald LJ. Treatment of intra-alveolar root fractures. Gen Dent 1988;33:412.
9. Soporowski NJ, Allred EN, Needleman HL. Luxation injuries of primary anterior teeth: prognosis and related correlates. Pediatr Dent 1994;16:96.
10. Crona-Larsson G, Bjarnason S, Noren JG. Effect of luxation injuries on permanent teeth. Endod Dent Traumatol 1991;7:199.
11. Andreason JO. Injuries to the supporting bone. In: Andreason JO, Andreason FM, editors. Textbook and color atlas of traumatic injuries to the teeth. 3rd edition. Copenhagen (Denmark): Munksgaard; 1994. p. 427–53.

12. Miloro M, Leathers RD, Gowans RE. Management of alveolar and dental fractures. In: Peterson's principles of oral and maxillofacial surgery. 2nd edition. Hamilton, Ontario (CA): BC Becker; 2004. p. 383.

13. Fonseca RJ, Walker RV, Betts NJ, et al. Oral and maxillofacial trauma. 3rd edition. Elsevier; 2004. p. 427–77.

14. Abubaker AO, Giglio JA, Strauss RA. Diagnosis and management of dentoveolar injuries. OMS knowledge update, vol. 3. American Association of Oral and Maxillofacial Surgeons; 2001. Trauma section, p. 29.

Management of Facial Bite Wounds

Panagiotis K. Stefanopoulos, DDS, LT COL (DC)[a],*,
Andromache D. Tarantzopoulou, DDS[b]

KEYWORDS

- Bite wound • Facial injury • Animal bite
- Human bite • Soft-tissue infection

Bite wounds have always been considered complex injuries contaminated with a unique polymicrobial inoculum. Because wounds of the extremities constitute the majority of bite cases, most relevant studies have focused on the wound infection rate in these areas. However, a substantial subset of dog, cat, and human bites, each in the order of 15%, are located on the face,[1–4] where fear of potential disfigurement is an overriding concern and the associated psychological consequences can be devastating.[5]

Although a wide range of mammals have been implicated in facial bite injuries,[6–13] the majority of these injuries are inflicted by dogs.[6,9,12,13] It is estimated that there are 44,000 facial injuries from dog bites affecting children each year in the United States.[3–5,9,12,14–22] Not surprisingly, facial injuries predominate in those dog-bite casualties requiring hospitalization.[14,20]

For half a century, oral and maxillofacial surgeons have remained in the forefront of the surgical treatment of these injuries, with expertise in the pathogenic oral flora, due to their dental background.[12,23–27] Nevertheless, certain aspects of therapy remain amenable to personal opinions and clinical impressions.[18,28] The aim of this article is to discuss these issues in the general context of bite-wound management (**Box 1**), including the role of prophylactic antibiotics and the possible limitations of the general axiom of primary closure.

WOUND CHARACTERISTICS

Animal bites can result in three main types of soft tissue trauma, namely punctures, lacerations, and avulsions, with or without an actual tissue defect.[14,23,29–31] The typical

A version of this article originally appeared in Stefanopoulos PK. Management of Facial Bite Wounds. Oral Max Surg Clin North Am 2009;21:247–57.

[a] Hellenic Army, Department of Oral and Maxillofacial Surgery, 401 Army Hospital, Athens, Greece

[b] Department of Periodontology and Implant Biology, Dental School, Aristotle University of Thessaloniki, Thessaloniki, Greece

* Corresponding author. 88 Pontou Street, Goudi, Athens 11527, Greece.

E-mail address: pstefanopoulos@yahoo.com (P.K. Stefanopoulos).

Dent Clin N Am 53 (2009) 691–705
doi:10.1016/j.cden.2009.08.005

dental.theclinics.com

Box 1
Controversial topics in the management of facial bite wounds

- Selection of solution for wound irrigation
- Irrigation of puncture wounds
- Role of antibiotic prophylaxis
- Selection of antimicrobial agent(s)
- Cutoff time for primary closure

---

dog bite results in a combination of torn tissues and adjacent punctures, the so-called "hole-and-tear" effect (**Fig. 1**).[32] Some degree of crush injury is also present in most bite wounds, including those from humans, due to the dynamics of the bite.[27,33] Dog bites of the face are located mostly on the lips, nose, or cheeks.[12,14,15,18,21,34–36] Human bites notably tend to involve the ear,[24,31,37,38] although the lower lip is also prominently involved.[24,39–43]

Bite wounds inflicted to the head and neck region by large animals can present in a more serious fashion.[7,10,11] Large dog attacks can result in life-threatening or even fatal injuries because of airway compromise, exsanguination, or craniocerebral trauma.[22,44–46] Furthermore, dog bites can impart enough energy to the facial skeleton to cause structural damage, especially in children.[15,29,46,47]

OVERVIEW OF MICROBIOLOGY

The importance of the indigenous oral bacteria in bite-wound infections is substantiated by the high isolation rates (>50% of cases) of *Pasteurella* spp from dog and cat bites,[33,48,49] and viridans streptococci, especially *Streptococcus anginosus*, from human bites.[30] There are also corresponding figures for oral anaerobes, including *Fusobacterium nucleatum*, *Bacteroides*, *Prevotella*, and *Porphyromonas* spp.[12,30,49] It should be appreciated, however, that almost any oral organism can become a potential pathogen under the right circumstances.[50]

Consistent with the heterogeneity observed between feline and canine oropharyngeal *Pasteurella* strains,[51] *P canis* biotype 1 is the predominant isolate from dog bites, whereas *P multocida* subspecies *multocida* and *septica* have been isolated much more

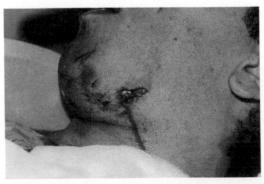

Fig. 1. Dog-bite wound of the face with scratches, punctures, and laceration ("hole-and-tear" effect).

frequently from cat bites.[49,52] Streptococci and staphylococci are the next most common aerobic isolates.[49,53] Potentially invasive aerobic organisms isolated from domestic animal bites include *Bergeyella* (*Weeksella*) *zoohelcum* and *Capnocytophaga canimorsus*, the latter associated with fulminant systemic infections in immunocompromised hosts, usually after a dog bite.[49,54–56]

Staphylococci are also commonly isolated from human bites.[30,53,57] *Eikenella corrodens*, a normal inhabitant of the human oral cavity, appears to have a unique association with human bites, having been recovered from about 30% of cases.[30] Other fastidious gram-negative organisms, such as *Haemophilus* spp and enteric gram-negative rods, have been found less frequently.[30,57] Oral as well as environmental fungi may also contaminate bite wounds.[54] *Candida* spp have been isolated from 8% of infected human bites, but their pathogenic role remains unclear.[30]

Bites can also impart systemic bacterial and viral infections, including classic zoonoses.[58] Human bites can be the source of the hepatitis B and C virus, and possibly HIV transmission, as well as syphilis.[27,59] Rabies remains the most dreaded of all animal bite-wound infections, which should be especially considered when bites from bats, raccoons, or foxes are encountered.[27,59,60]

RISK FACTORS FOR WOUND INFECTION

Facial bite wounds generally display low infection rates, commonly attributed to the rich blood supply of the area.[2,18,55,61] Dog bites on the face are usually considered to be at moderate risk for infection when compared with other types of mammalian bites,[33] especially those inflicted by cats,[6,12] which harbor the more toxic *P multocida* organisms.[52] Furthermore, dog-bite wounds seen within 3 hours of injury rarely contain more than 10^5 bacteria per gram of tissue, while human bites usually exceed this critical level[62] because of higher bacterial counts in saliva.[63]

Significant delays–beyond 6 to 12 hours–in seeking medical attention increase the likelihood of infection.[12,22,31,38,39,64–66] Victims of bites to the face are more likely to present in time for prompt wound care than do other bite victims, because of concern about possible scarring.[16,21] However, long delays may be encountered with facial bites, due to alcohol intoxication of the victim[31] or transport from remote areas.[42] Furthermore, prolonged exposure of the wound to bacterial contamination can affect the therapeutic efficacy of antibiotics.[64,67] Unfortunately, no study has controlled for the time from wounding to antibiotic treatment.[68]

Puncture wounds, typically inflicted by the slender feline teeth, are associated with high infection rates because they involve deep inoculation of pathogens.[12,44,69,70] Crush injuries, on the other hand, can precipitate infection with significantly lower bacterial counts because of the resultant tissue ischemia.[57,64,69,71] However, due to the inevitable cartilage exposure, avulsion injuries of the ear or nose inflicted by humans have the highest incidence of infection following facial bite wounds, according to reports.[38]

CLINICAL EVALUATION

With extensive head or neck injury, life-preserving emergency procedures take precedence;[11,22,27,28,46,59,70,72] cervical immobilization should also be considered.[22] Otherwise, there is time to obtain the necessary information about the incident as well as about the general condition of the patient.[44,70]

When there is a possibility of involvement of underlying specialized structures, early diagnosis is essential. Eyelid lacerations require careful evaluation to rule out penetrating injury to the globe or interruption of the lacrimal drainage system.[59,73,74]

Radiographic examination of the adjacent facial or cranial bones is indicated when a fracture is suspected.[15,22,75,76] A proposed classification of facial bite wounds,[15,77] based on extent, appears in **Table 1**.

The wound should be assessed for signs of infection, including redness, swelling, or discharge. These signs tend to be more obvious with older wounds than with fresh ones.[12,49] Fever is generally unlikely.[44,48,78,79] P multocida organisms are associated with a rapid onset of infection,[52,78] whereas when the latency period is more than 24 hours, staphylococci, streptococci, or anaerobes are more likely etiologic agents.[22,49,72,79] Cultures are most useful in case initial antibiotic therapy fails.[69]

Bite wounds are considered tetanus-prone,[11,59,72] so appropriate immunization should be administered if the patient has had fewer than three doses of tetanus toxoid or more than 5 years have passed since the last dose.[80–82] Rabies prophylaxis should be based on the local prevalence of the disease, the biting species, and the circumstances surrounding the incident.[44,50,58,59,79,82]

Superficial bite wounds can be treated in the outpatient setting, whereas patients with more serious injuries (types III and IV) should be hospitalized and treated in the operating room. For children whose wounds require surgical care, hospitalization should be considered because they may be uncooperative under local anesthesia.[15,77] Signs of systemic toxicity, rapidly advancing cellulitis, or infection despite oral antibiotic therapy constitute other indications for hospitalization.[56,76] Most adults with uncomplicated bite wounds (type II) can be discharged after wound repair with instructions for follow-up.[77]

LOCAL WOUND CARE

As with any laceration, the mainstays of wound care are irrigation and removal of any necrotic tissue.[58,72,75] However, common practices, such as cleansing with soap or scrubbing,[44,58] are best reserved for high-risk wounds. Irrigation is essential in preventing infection because it removes debris and microorganisms;[59,61,71,72,75,83,84] wounds difficult to irrigate thoroughly, such as punctures, are twice as likely to become infected.[85] Manual irrigation with a 19-gauge catheter on a 30- to 60-mL syringe delivers a pressure range between 5 and 8 psi, considered optimal for appropriate decontamination.[83,84,86,87] Continuous irrigation seems to be just as effective as pulsatile lavage.[86] However, sustained high-pressure irrigation should be avoided in

Table 1	
Classification of facial bite injuries	

Type	Clinical Findings
I	Superficial injury without muscle involvement
IIA	Deep injury with muscle involvement
IIB	Full-thickness injury of the cheek or lip with oral mucosal involvement (through-and-through wound)
IIIA	Deep injury with tissue defect (complete avulsion)
IIIB	Deep avulsive injury exposing nasal or auricular cartilage
IVA	Deep injury with severed facial nerve and/or parotid duct
IVB	Deep injury with concomitant bone fracture

From Stefanopoulos PK, Tarantzopoulou AD. Facial bite wounds: management update. Int J Oral Maxillofac Surg 2005;34:469. (Modified from Lackmann GM, Draf W, Isselstein G, et al. Surgical treatment of facial dog bite injuries in children. J Craniomaxillofac Surg 1992;20:85; with permission.)

areas containing loose areolar tissue, such as the eyelids or children's cheeks, because such irrigation may cause tissue disruption and excessive edema.[72] In general, 250 to 500 mL of solution provides an adequate cleansing effect for most facial bite wounds.[75,88] Although irrigation of puncture wounds remains controversial because of the inherent difficulties in proper drainage,[72] most investigators also use pressure irrigation for these wounds, taking care to allow escape of the fluid (**Box 2**).[12,44,88] Incising the puncture to promote irrigation[27] is not recommended, however, as it causes unnecessary scarring.[16]

Normal saline is the fluid of choice for irrigation, according to many experts.[16,22,44,72,75,76,84,86,88] A 1% povidone-iodine solution also has been recommended for irrigation of bite wounds because this solution provides an optimal therapeutic balance between bactericidal capacity and tissue toxicity associated with iodine-containing formulations.[33,69,79,87] However, when used under pressure for wound decontamination, saline has compared favorably with 1% povidone-iodine solution and other less commonly used alternatives.[89,90] Moreover, even if povidone-iodine or another antiseptic solution is used as an irrigant, copious rinsing with normal saline should follow to minimize the risk of cytotoxicity.[12,15,27]

Surgical debridement is a common clinical practice in bite-wound management[16,37,40,88] because it significantly decreases the likelihood of infection.[57,85] However, debridement of facial wounds should be kept to a minimum so as to avoid sacrifice of tissue that has a good chance to survive,[12,34,38,56] particularly in landmark areas such as the vermilion border of the lips, the nasolabial fold, and the eyebrows (**Box 2**).[25,42,59,75]

Box 2
Treatment protocol for common facial bite wounds

1. Skin preparation; anesthesia
2. Pressure irrigation; irrigation of puncture wounds
3. Resection of skin tags
4. Removal of visible foreign particles
5. Suturing (exceptions listed below)
6. Consideration of tetanus prophylaxis
7. Follow-up within 24 to 48 hours

Also recommended:

Normal saline irrigation (1% povidone-iodine should be reserved for grossly contaminated wounds)

Antibiotic prophylaxis

Culture of problematic wounds (failure to respond to initial antibiotic therapy or presence of serious infection)

Not recommended:

Routine debridement (if attempted, it should not exceed 1 mm of tissue)

Suturing in the presence of overt infection, gross edema, foreign bodies, or visible contamination (consider delayed closure)

Culture of fresh uninfected wounds, because it depicts the polymicrobial flora of the wound rather than the causative organisms of any subsequent infection

SURGICAL TREATMENT

Primary wound closure is the treatment of choice for all uninfected facial bite lacerations seen within 24 hours, as well as for many avulsion injuries, because this obtains the most favorable esthetic result.[12,16–18,26–28,34–36,39–43,59,64,75,91] Subcutaneous sutures should be used sparingly, however, because they can act as foreign bodies and precipitate infection.[27,59] By contrast, deep puncture wounds should be left open, particularly when inflicted by cats.[27,59]

In the study of Maimaris and Quinton,[65] 1 of 27 sutured wounds in the face became infected compared with none of the 14 wounds left open, a difference considered both insignificant and acceptable in view of the better cosmetic result achieved with suturing. Several other studies have confirmed the low risk associated with suturing of facial bite wounds,[2,41,88,92] although in some studies increased infection rates were found both with dog bites[12,46] and human bites.[38]

For uncomplicated bite wounds presenting beyond the "golden 24-hour period," primary closure is controversial.[93] In these cases, delayed closure is a time-honored practice.[38,71,84] This implies a waiting period of 4 to 5 days before definitive wound closure, during which time the wound is kept open, usually with moist gauze dressings providing drainage, while edema is allowed to subside.[94,95] Antibiotics can be administered to further diminish the risk of infection.[38,87,95]

Other surgeons, however, prefer to proceed with primary repair of late-presenting wounds to achieve a less noticeable scar, although this approach may increase the risk for infection.[16,39,96] This approach has been substantiated by studies suggesting that primary closure of facial human bites can be undertaken with an acceptable risk within 48 hours and even as late as the fourth day after the incident.[40,42,57] However, these studies included mainly low-risk wounds (ie, avulsion type rather than punctures or crush injuries),[97] most of them located on the lips, which are very resistant to the development of infection.

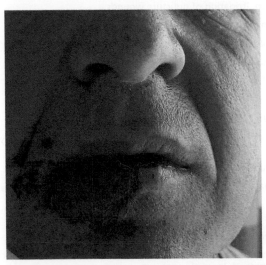

Fig. 2. Full-thickness dog-bite avulsion injury of the lower lip 1 day after an unsuccessful attempt at simple (non-microsurgical) reattachment in another hospital. Note absence of infection. The defect was later reconstructed with flap surgery by a plastic surgeon. (*Courtesy of* Kyriakos Kapagerides, MD, LT COL.)

Avulsion bite wounds can pose reconstructive challenges if direct closure is not possible. Attempts to reattach avulsed parts are usually doomed to fail (**Fig. 2**).[35,37,38] In these cases, local skin flaps or composite grafts should be considered, depending on the area involved.[16,18,37,39,41,46,57] Microsurgical replantation has become the standard operation in some centers,[12,98] yet it remains technically demanding.[99] Recently, an extensive soft tissue defect of the face due to a severe dog bite was reconstructed with partial face transplantation.[100]

The presence of overt infection normally precludes suturing the wound. Options include secondary healing with subsequent revision surgery, delayed closure (**Box 2**),[24,38,39] or primary closure with insertion of a drain.[12] Successful immediate primary closure has been reported after debridement with proteolytic agents.[26]

ANTIBIOTIC TREATMENT

Antibiotic administration for bite wounds can be either prophylactic or therapeutic.[12,101] In the presence of established infection or any underlying predisposing condition, antibiotic therapy is indicated. However, it remains unclear whether otherwise healthy patients with fresh clinically uninfected wounds benefit from prophylactic antibiotic administration.[18,55,101] Even in these cases, however, antibiotic therapy may actually be therapeutic if enough time has elapsed for bacterial proliferation to reach a level that can result in the development of infection.[11,58,66]

On the basis of figures from a meta-analysis of prophylactic antibiotics for dog-bite wounds,[102] Callaham[67] calculated that as many as 26 patients must be treated with oral antibiotics to prevent 1 infection. Consistently, infection rates in the order of 4% have been reported with primary repair of facial dog-bite wounds without the use of antibiotics.[65,88] On the other hand, with two notable exceptions,[34,46] equally good results have been obtained when antibiotics were administrated.[35,36] Obviously, little evidence supports the value of prophylactic antibiotics in the treatment of dog-bite wounds,[91] although the type of wound, the particular location, and any additional contamination may necessitate antibiotic coverage.[27]

Consensus exists regarding antibiotic prophylaxis for cat-bite wounds because of their high-risk character.[2,12,44,59,70,76,79] Patients with human bites are also serious candidates for antibiotic prophylaxis. Limited evidence suggests that antibiotics for human bites of the face may result in infection rates as low as 2.5%.[37] Furthermore, in a recent study,[38] mainly dealing with high-risk avulsion injuries of the ear, failure to receive at least 48 hours of prophylactic intravenous antibiotics was associated with an increased infection risk following primary closure.

In view of the incomplete debridement permitted on the face,[95] most investigators favor antibiotic prophylaxis for facial bite wounds[12,18,20,35,43,44,46,58,60,81,91] because even low infection rates can seriously compromise cosmetic outcome, especially in children.[77] Furthermore, it has been suggested that primary closure may also increase the risk of infection,[33,92] thus further justifying prophylactic antibiotics in such cases.[56,60,76] Because the indications for antibiotics do not correlate well with the severity of injury,[46] prophylaxis is generally recommended for all bites penetrating the skin.[12,58,77]

For most terrestrial mammal bites, the choice of antibiotics is based on experience with dog, cat, and human bites.[11,50,55,82] Furthermore, because *E corrodens* exhibits similar susceptibility patterns to *Pasteurella* organisms, identical regimens are used for human and most animal bites.[82] Traditional approaches involve selective coverage for the most likely pathogens, including staphylococci, streptococci, and either *Pasteurella* spp for dog and cat bites or *E corrodens*, and oral anaerobes for human bites.

Most of these bacteria are susceptible to penicillin, but many strains of S aureus and Prevotella produce β-lactamase. Thus appropriate regimens should include combinations of penicillin with an antistaphylococcal penicillin or a first-generation cephalosporin,[15,68,70,79] possibly with the addition of metronidazole.

According to current recommendations, amoxicillin/clavulanate is the antimicrobial agent of choice for prophylaxis of bite wounds[27,35,44,59,81,82,91,93,101,103] as it remains active against most animal and human bite-wound isolates.[22,30,49,58,104,105] Few clinical trials have examined the use of amoxicillin/clavulanate in bite cases[66] and reports have appeared noting the failure of amoxicillin/clavulanate in some relevant situations. [92] However, in the series of Kesting and Colleagues,[12] none of the patients who received amoxicillin/clavulanate developed infection, and others have also reported good results with this regimen.[35]

In case of allergy to penicillin, available alternatives include cefuroxime axetil for patients with mild allergy, whereas those with a history of a severe reaction can receive doxycycline[44,81] or a combination of clindamycin with either a fluoroquinolone or trimethoprim-sulfamethoxazole (for children).[56,82,103] Cefuroxime axetil is a recommended alternative for cat-bite wounds,[77,103] but clinical failures have been reported.[106] Moxifloxacin has shown good activity against most bite-wound pathogens, with the exception of most fusobacteria,[58,104,105] and is useful for adult patients allergic to penicillin.[82,106] Azithromycin is probably the most appropriate choice for penicillin-allergic pregnant women or children, for whom tetracyclines, fluoroquinolones, and sulfa compounds are contraindicated.[56,77,82]

For the treatment of established infection, the same basic antibiotic regimens should be followed, except that they should be administered intravenously.[59] Combinations of a β-lactam/β-lactamase inhibitor, such as ampicillin/sulbactam or ticarcillin/clavulanate, moxifloxacin or cefoxitin (because of its anti-anaerobic activity), are all excellent choices;[58,81,103,107] most other second- or third-generation cephalosporins require the addition of an anti-anaerobic agent.[107] The in vitro activity of the previously mentioned agents against most common bite-wound pathogens is listed in **Table 2**, and recommended regimens for prophylaxis are outlined in **Table 3**.

The typical course for antibiotic prophylaxis is 3 to 5 days.[11,55,107] The duration of therapeutic antibiotics varies, depending on the severity of the infection. Most cases of cellulitis require a total of 10 to 14 days.[22,55,56] If cultures were obtained, specific antimicrobial therapy should be based on the culture results.[56] Cases of associated fractures should be treated according to the "therapeutic" rather than the "prophylactic" schedule.

DISCUSSION

Undoubtedly, high-pressure irrigation has a crucial role in the conversion of the contaminated (or even dirty) bite wound into a clean-contaminated environment suitable for subsequent primary closure. Routine use of normal saline is recommended on the premise that emphasis should be placed on the mechanical effect rather than on any antibacterial activity of a more potent solution, which on such a complex wound would be a potential irritant or at best only temporarily effective (see **Box 2**). The use of antiseptic solutions also tends to cause a false sense of security and thus encourages breaching of the treatment protocol. Debridement, if necessary, should not be overzealous. Precise realignment of irregular wound edges is always rewarding in the face and should be preferred to their excision.

Authoritative opinion has pulled back somewhat from previous overconfidence that the vascularity of the face and scalp consistently leads to a favorable outcome for

Table 2
Antimicrobial activity of selected oral agents against common bite-wound pathogens

Agent	Pasteurella Multocida	Staphylococcus Aureus	Streptococcus Spp	Streptococcus "Milleri" (S Anginosus)	Eikenella Corrodens	Prevotella Spp	Fusobacterium Nucleatum
Penicillin	+	−	+	+	+	±	+
Amoxicillin/ clavulanate	+	+	+	+	+	+	+
Cefuroxime	+	+	+	+	+	−	−
Doxycycline	+	+	±	−	±	+	+
Erythromycin	−	+	±	±	−	+	−
Azithromycin	+	+	+	+	±	+	±
Ciprofloxacin	+	+	±	0	+	0	0
Moxifloxacin	+	+	+	+	+	+	−
TMP-SMX	+	+	+	+	+	0	0
Clindamycin	0	+	+	+	0	+	+

Key: +, good activity; ±, intermediate activity, probably clinically useful; −, poor activity, clinically unpredictable; 0, no activity.

Abbreviation: TMP-SMX, trimethoprim-sulfamethoxazole.

Data from Goldstein EJC. Outpatient management of dog and cat bite wounds. Family Practice Recertification 2000;22:67–86; Goldstein EJC, Citron DM, Hudspeth M, et al. In vitro activity of Bay 12-8039, a new 8-methoxyquinolone, compared with the activities of 11 other oral antimicrobial agents against 390 aerobic and anaerobic bacteria isolated from human and animal bite wound skin and soft tissue infections in humans. Antimicrobial Agents Chemother 1997;41:1552–7; and Goldstein EJC, Citron DM, Merriam CV, et al. Comparative in vitro activity of faropenem and 11 other antimicrobial agents against 405 aerobic and anaerobic pathogens isolated from skin and soft tissue infections from animal and human bites. J Antimicrob Chemother 2002;50:411–20.

Table 3
Antimicrobial prophylaxis for common facial bite wounds

Patient	Primary Regimen	Alternative Regimens/Allergy
Adult	Amoxicillin/clavulanate	Clindamycin plus ciprofloxacin Cefuroxime axetil Doxycycline Moxifloxacin Azithromycin
Child	Amoxicillin/clavulanate	Clindamycin plus TMP-SMX Azithromycin
Pregnant	Amoxicillin/clavulanate	Azithromycin

Abbreviation: TMP-SMX, trimethoprim-sulfamethoxazole.

such bite wounds. Realizing that these wounds actually carry a significant risk for infection, influential investigators now recommend antibiotic prophylaxis. This is also the opinion of the author. Two additional factors pertaining to the face can render the management of bite wounds in this area problematic. The first is a substantial risk of occult oral communication with dog-bite injuries of the cheek because of the nature of the dog's occlusion. The second is the presence of the relatively avascular buccal fat pad, which is very developed in children and, once exposed, does not resist infection well. Thus, in cases of deep bites to the cheek, especially in children, after careful exploration and irrigation, antibiotic "prophylaxis" should be started as soon as possible, usually with the first dose administered intravenously.

Determining when to make the repair can be tricky. This is especially true in cases presenting late at night. In such cases, the clinician may prefer a delay to a time when the best expertise is available and operating conditions more suitable. However, delay might make eventual repair more difficult. On the one hand, evidence suggests that some linear lacerations can be safely repaired under antibiotic coverage even when presenting several days after the injury. On the other hand, severely crushed or mangled wounds, besides being at increased risk for infection, tend to become very edematous within hours. Delayed primary closure is indicated in the latter cases to avoid dehiscence because of approximation under tension. Along with experts in the field,[108] the author believes that the decision about timing of repair should be based not so much on the age of the wound as on its appearance.

Finally, as to the proper setting for surgical intervention, most victims with uncomplicated injuries can receive treatment as outpatients. However, even with the most cooperative patients, inadequate assistance or lighting in the crowded emergency department can be very frustrating and may result in compromise with the principles of facial reconstruction. Therefore, it is preferable to treat even type II injuries in the operating room, if possible, to allow for proper irrigation and meticulous repair of the wound.[109]

SUMMARY

Primary closure is the standard of care for most facial bite wounds, preceded by proper wound irrigation and debridement, where indicated. Administration of antibiotics, preferably on admission, is advisable for all injuries requiring suturing; clean linear lacerations, treated within 3 hours after injury, are possible exceptions. Depending on the clinical appearance of the lesion, patients presenting beyond the first 24 hours should be treated with delayed closure. This option should especially be contemplated for those wounds with gross contamination or with crushed, ischemic, or edematous edges. Serious injuries with bone involvement should be treated according to established protocols. In all cases, clinical judgment should be used and close follow-up is recommended to reduce future complications.

ACKNOWLEDGMENTS

The senior author wishes to thank Professor Michael L. Callaham, MD, for his kind suggestions, and Miss Martha Petromihelaki, for her constant help with the literature search.

REFERENCES

1. Marr JS, Beck AM, Lugo JA. An epidemiologic study of the human bite. Public Health Rep 1979;94:514–21.
2. Dire DJ. Cat bite wounds: risk factors for infection. Ann Emerg Med 1991;20:973–9.
3. Borud LJ, Friedman DW. Dog bites in New York City. Plast Reconstr Surg 2000; 106:989–90.
4. Centers for Disease Control and Prevention. Nonfatal dog-bite related injuries treated in hospital emergency departments—United States, 2001. MMWR Morb Mortal Wkly Rep 2003;52(26):605–10.
5. Schalamon J, Ainoedhofer H, Singer G, et al. Analysis of dog bites in children who are younger than 17 years. Pediatrics 2006;117:374–9.
6. Aghababian RV, Conte JE. Mammalian bite wounds. Ann Emerg Med 1980;9: 79–83.
7. Govila A, Rao GS, James JH. Primary reconstruction of a major loss of lower jaw by an animal bite using a "rib sandwich" pectoralis major island flap. Br J Plast Surg 1989;42:101–3.
8. Ogunbodede EO, Arotiba JT. Camel bite injuries of the orofacial region: report of a case. J Oral Maxillofac Surg 1997;55:1174–6.
9. Matter HC, The Sentinel Working Group. The epidemiology of bite and scratch injuries by vertebrate animals in Switzerland. Eur J Epidemiol 1998;14:483–90.
10. Bahram R, Burke JE, Lanzi GL. Head and neck injury from a leopard attack: case report and review of the literature. J Oral Maxillofac Surg 2004;62:247–9.
11. Freer L. North American wild mammalian injuries. Emerg Med Clin North Am 2004;22:445–73.
12. Kesting MR, Hölzle F, Pox C, et al. Animal bite injuries to the head: 132 cases. Br J Oral Maxillofac Surg 2006;44:235–9.
13. MacBean C, Taylor DMcD, Ashby K. Animal and human bite injuries in Victoria, 1998–2004. Med J Aust 2007;186:38–40.
14. Karlson TA. The incidence of facial injuries from dog bites. JAMA 1984;251: 3265–7.
15. Lackmann G-M, Draf W, Isselstein G, et al. Surgical treatment of facial dog bite injuries in children. J Craniomaxillofac Surg 1992;20(2):81–6.
16. Hallock GG. Dog bites of the face with tissue loss. J Craniomaxillofac Trauma 1996;2:49–55.
17. Scheithauer MO, Rettinger G. Bißverletzungen im Kopf-Halsbereich. HNO 1997; 45:891–7.
18. Kountakis SE, Chamblee SA, Maillard AAJ, et al. Animal bites to the head and neck. Ear Nose Throat J 1998;77:216–20.
19. Weiss HB, Friedman DI, Coben JH. Incidence of dog bite injuries treated in emergency departments. JAMA 1998;279:51–3.

20. Kahn A, Bauche P, Lamoureux J. Child victims of dog bites treated in emergency departments: a prospective survey. Eur J Pediatr 2003;162:254–8.
21. Van Eeckhout GPA, Wylock P. Dog bites: an overview. European Journal of Plastic Surgery 2005;28:233–8.
22. Morgan M, Palmer J. Dog bites. BMJ 2007;334:413–7.
23. Laskin DM, Donohue WB. Treatment of human bites of the lip. J Oral Surg 1958; 16:236–42.
24. Tomasetti BJ, Walker L, Gormley MB, et al. Human bites of the face. J Oral Surg 1979;37:565–8.
25. Ruskin JD, Laney TJ, Wendt SV, et al. Treatment of mammalian bite wounds of the maxillofacial region. J Oral Maxillofac Surg 1993;51:174–6.
26. Baurmash HD, Monto M. Delayed healing human bite wounds of the orofacial area managed with immediate primary closure: treatment rationale. J Oral Maxillofac Surg 2005;63:1391–7.
27. Cunningham LL Jr, Robinson FG, Haug RH, et al. Management of human and animal bites. In: Fonseca RJ, Walker RV, Betts NJ, editors. Oral and maxillofacial trauma. 3rd edition. St Louis (MO): Elsevier Saunders; 2005. p. 843–62.
28. Leach J. Proper handling of sift tissue in the acute phase. Facial Plast Surg 2001;17:227–38.
29. Tu AH, Girotto JA, Singh N, et al. Facial fractures from dog bite injuries. Plast Reconstr Surg 2002;109:1259–65.
30. Talan DA, Abrahamian FM, Moran GJ, et al. Clinical presentation and bacteriologic analysis of infected human bites in patients presenting to emergency departments. Clin Infect Dis 2003;37:1481–9.
31. Henry FP, Purcell EM, Eadie PA. The human bite injury: a clinical audit and discussion regarding the management of this alcohol fuelled phenomenon. Emerg Med J 2007;24:455–8.
32. De Munnynck K, Van de Voorde W. Forensic approach of fatal dog attacks: a case report and literature review. Int J Legal Med 2002;116:295–300.
33. Dire DJ, Hogan DE, Riggs MW. A prospective evaluation of risk factors for infections from dog-bite wounds. Acad Emerg Med 1994;1:258–66.
34. Palmer J, Rees M. Dog bites of the face: a 15 year review. Br J Plast Surg 1983; 36:315–8.
35. Javaid M, Feldberg L, Gipson M. Primary repair of dog bites to the face: 40 cases. J R Soc Med 1998;91:414–6 B.
36. Mcheik JN, Vergnes P, Bondonny JM. Treatment of facial dog bite injuries in children: a retrospective study. J Pediatr Surg 2000;35:580–3.
37. Earley MJ, Bardsley AF. Human bites: a review. Br J Plast Surg 1984;37: 458–62.
38. Stierman KL, Lloyd KM, De Luca-Pytell D, et al. Treatment and outcome of human bites in the head and neck. Otolaryngol Head Neck Surg 2003;128: 795–801.
39. Losken HW, Auchincloss JA. Human bites of the lip. Clin Plast Surg 1984;11:773–5.
40. Venter THJ. Human bites of the face. S Afr Med J 1988;74:277–9.
41. Uchendu BO. Primary closure of human bite losses of the lip. Plast Reconstr Surg 1992;90:841–5.
42. Donkor P, Bankas DO. A study of primary closure of human bite injuries to the face. J Oral Maxillofac Surg 1997;55:479–81.
43. Chidzonga MM. Human bites of the face. S Afr Med J 1998;88:150–2.
44. Goldstein EJC. Outpatient management of dog and cat bite wounds. Family Practice Recertification 2000;22:67–86.

45. Calkins CM, Bensard DD, Partrick DA, et al. Life-threatening dog attacks: a devastating combination of penetrating and blunt injuries. J Pediatr Surg 2001;36:1115–7.
46. Mitchell RB, Nañez G, Wagner JD, et al. Dog bites of the scalp, face, and neck in children. Laryngoscope 2003;113:492–5.
47. Fourie L, Cartilidge D. Fracture of the maxilla following dog bite to the face. Injury 1995;26:61–2.
48. Goldstein EJC. New horizons in the bacteriology, antimicrobial susceptibility and therapy of animal bite wounds. J Med Microbiol 1998;47:95–7 [editorial].
49. Talan DA, Citron DM, Abrahamian FM, et al. Bacteriologic analysis of infected dog and cat bites. N Engl J Med 1999;340:85–92.
50. Goldstein EJC. Current concepts on animal bites: bacteriology and therapy. Curr Clin Top Infect Dis 1999;19:99–111.
51. Holst E, Rollof J, Larsson L, et al. Characterization and distribution of Pasteurella species recovered from infected humans. J Clin Microbiol 1992;30:2984–7.
52. Westling K, Farra A, Cars B, et al. Cat bite wound infections: a prospective clinical and microbiological study at three emergency wards in Stockholm, Sweden. J Infect 2006;53:403–7.
53. Brook I. Microbiology of human and animal bite wounds in children. Pediatr Infect Dis J 1987;6:29–32.
54. Barnham M. Once bitten twice shy: the microbiology of bites. Rev Med Microbiol 1991;2:31–6.
55. Goldstein EJC. Bite wounds and infection. Clin Infect Dis 1992;14:633–40.
56. Abrahamian FM. Dog bites: bacteriology, management, and prevention. Curr Infect Dis Rep 2000;2:446–53.
57. Agrawal K, Mishra S, Panda KN. Primary reconstruction of major human bite wounds of the face. Plast Reconstr Surg 1992;90:394–8.
58. Brook I. Management of human and animal bite wounds: an overview. Adv Skin Wound Care 2005;18:197–203.
59. Fleisher GR. The management of bite wounds. N Engl J Med 1999;340:138–40 [editorial].
60. Hoff GL, Brawley J, Johnson K. Companion animal issues and the physician. South Med J 1999;92:651–9.
61. Callaham ML. Treatment of common dog bites: infection risk factors. JACEP 1978;7:83–7.
62. Krizek TJ, Robson MC. Evolution of quantitative bacteriology in wound management. Am J Surg 1975;130:579–84.
63. von Troil-Lindén B, Torkko H, Alaluusua S, et al. Salivary levels of suspected periodontal pathogens in relation to periodontal status and treatment. J Dent Res 1995;74:1789–93.
64. Edlich RF, Spengler MD, Rodeheaver GT, et al. Emergency department management of mammalian bites. Emerg Med Clin North Am 1986;4:595–604.
65. Maimaris C, Quinton DN. Dog-bite lacerations: a controlled trial of primary wound closure. Arch Emerg Med 1988;5:156–61.
66. Brakenbury PH, Muwanga C. A comparative double blind study of amoxicillin/clavulanate vs placebo in the prevention of infection after animal bites. Arch Emerg Med 1989;6:251–6.
67. Callaham M. Prophylactic antibiotics in dog bite wounds: nipping at the heels of progress. Ann Emerg Med 1994;23:577–9 [editorial].

68. Callaham M. Controversies in antibiotic choices for bite wounds. Ann Emerg Med 1988;17:1321–30.
69. Callaham ML. Human and animal bites. Top Emerg Med 1982;4:1–13.
70. Weber EJ. Mammalian bites. In: Marx JA, editor. Rosen's emergency medicine: concepts and clinical practice. 6th edition. St Louis (MO): Mosby; 2006. p. 882–92.
71. Lieblich SE, Topazian RG. Infection in the patient with maxillofacial trauma. In: Fonseca RJ, Walker RV, Betts NJ, et al, editors. Oral and maxillofacial trauma. 3rd edition. St Louis (MO): Elsevier Saunders; 2005. p. 1109–30.
72. Capellan O, Hollander JE. Management of lacerations in the emergency department. Emerg Med Clin North Am 2003;21:205–31.
73. Botek AA, Goldberg SH. Management of eyelid dog bites. J Craniomaxillofac Trauma 1996;1:18–24.
74. Slonim CB. Dog bite-induced canalicular lacerations: a review of 17 cases. Ophthal Plast Reconstr Surg 1996;12:218–22.
75. Abubaker AO. Management of posttraumatic soft tissue infections. Oral Maxillofac Surg Clin North Am 2003;15:139–46.
76. Correira K. Managing dog, cat, and human bite wounds. J Am Acad Physician Assist 2003;16:28–37.
77. Stefanopoulos PK, Tarantzopoulou AD. Facial bite wounds: management update. Int J Oral Maxillofac Surg 2005;34:464–72.
78. Holm M, Tärnvik A. Hospitalization due to Pasteurella multocida–infected animal bite wounds: correlation with inadequate primary antibiotic medication. Scand J Infect Dis 2000;32:181–3.
79. Dire DJ. Animal bites. In: Singer AJ, Hollander JE, editors. Lacerations and acute wounds: an evidence-based guide. Philadelphia: F.A. Davis; 2003. p. 133–46.
80. Centers for Disease Control and Prevention. Advisory Committee on Immunization Practices. Preventing tetanus, diphtheria, and pertussis among adults: use of tetanus toxoid, reduced diphtheria toxoid and acellular pertussis vaccine. MMWR Recomm Rep 2006;55(RR17):1–37.
81. Bartlett JG. Johns Hopkins antibiotic guide: bite wounds. Available at: http://prod.hopkins-abxguide.org/diagnosis/soft_tissue/bite_wounds.
82. Moran GJ, Talan DA, Abrahamian FM. Antimicrobial prophylaxis for wounds and procedures in the emergency department. Infect Dis Clin North Am 2008;22:117–43.
83. Chisholm CD. Wound evaluation and cleansing. Emerg Med Clin North Am 1992;10:665–72.
84. Simon B, Hern HG Jr. Wound management principles. In: Marx JA, editor. Rosen's emergency medicine: concepts and clinical practice. 6th edition. Philadelphia: Mosby Elsevier; 2006. p. 842–57.
85. Callaham M. Prophylactic antibiotics in common dog bite wounds: a controlled study. Ann Emerg Med 1980;9:410–4.
86. Hollander JE, Singer AJ. Laceration management. Ann Emerg Med 1999;34:356–67.
87. Brancato JC. Minor wound preparation and irrigation. Up to date; version 16.1. Available at: www.uptodate.com.
88. Guy RJ, Zook EG. Successful treatment of acute head and neck dog bite wounds without antibiotics. Ann Plast Surg 1986;17:45–8.
89. Dire DJ, Welsh AP. A comparison of wound irrigation solutions used in the emergency department. Ann Emerg Med 1990;19:704–8.
90. Fernandez R, Griffiths R, Ussia C. Effectiveness of solutions, techniques and pressure in wound cleansing. The Joanna Briggs Institute Reports 2004;2:231–70.

91. Chaudhry MA, MacNamara AF, Clark S. Is the management of dog bite wounds evidence based? A postal survey and review of the literature. Eur J Emerg Med 2004;11:313–7.
92. Chen E, Hornig S, Shepherd SM, et al. Primary closure of mammalian bites. Acad Emerg Med 2000;7:157–61.
93. Vasconez HC. Soft tissue injuries. In: Goldwyn RM, Cohen MN, editors. The unfavorable result in plastic surgery: avoidance and treatment. 3rd edition. Philadelphia: Lippincott Williams & Wilkins; 2001. p. 453–65.
94. Dimick AR. Delayed wound closure: indications and techniques. Ann Emerg Med 1988;17:1303–4.
95. Dufresne CR, Manson PN. Pediatric facial injuries. In: Mathes SJ, editor. Plastic surgery. 2nd edition. Philadelphia: Saunders Elsevier; 2006. p. 381–462.
96. Eppley BL, Bhuller A. Principles of facial soft tissue injury repair. In: Ward Booth P, Eppley BL, Schmelzeisen R, editors. Maxillofacial trauma and esthetic facial reconstruction. Edinburgh: Churchill Livingstone; 2003. p. 107–20.
97. Ruskin JD. Discussion: a study of primary closure of human bite injuries to the face. J Oral Maxillofac Surg 1997;55:481–2.
98. Hussain G, Thomson S, Zielinski V. Nasal amputation due to human bite: microsurgical replantation. Aust N Z J Surg 1997;67:382–4.
99. Flores RL, Hazen A, Galiano RD, et al. Non-extremity replantation: the management of amputations of the facial parts and testicle. Clin Plast Surg 2007;34:197–210.
100. Devauchelle B, Badet L, Lengelé B, et al. First human face allograft: early report. Lancet 2006;368:203–9.
101. Nakamura Y, Daya M. Use of appropriate antimicrobials in wound management. Emerg Med Clin North Am 2007;25:159–76.
102. Cummings P. Antibiotics to prevent infection in patients with dog bite wounds: a meta-analysis of randomized trials. Ann Emerg Med 1994;23:535–40.
103. Gilbert DN, Moellering RC Jr, Eliopoulos GM, et al. The Sanford guide to antimicrobial therapy 2007. 37th edition. Sperryville (VA): Antimicrobial Therapy, Inc; 2007. p. 46–7.
104. Goldstein EJC, Citron DM, Hudspeth M, et al. In vitro activity of Bay 12–8039, a new 8-methoxyquinolone, compared to the activities of 11 other oral antimicrobial agents against 390 aerobic and anaerobic bacteria isolated from human and animal bite wound skin and soft tissue infections in humans. Antimicrobial Agents Chemother 1997;41:1552–7.
105. Goldstein EJC, Citron DM, Merriam CV, et al. Comparative in vitro activity of faropenem and 11 other antimicrobial agents against 405 aerobic and anaerobic pathogens isolated from skin and soft tissue infections from animal and human bites. J Antimicrob Chemother 2002;50:411–20.
106. Draenert R, Kunzelmann M, Roggenkamp A, et al. Infected cat-bite wound treated successfully with moxifloxacin after failure of parenteral cefuroxime and ciprofloxacin. Eur J Clin Microbiol Infect Dis 2005;24:288–90.
107. Stevens DL, Bisno AL, Chambers HF, et al. Practice guidelines for the diagnosis and management of skin and soft-tissue infections. Clin Infect Dis 2005;41:1373–406.
108. Cohen MN. Soft tissue injuries. In: Goldwyn RM, Cohen MN, editors. The unfavorable result in plastic surgery: avoidance and treatment. 3rd edition. Philadelphia: Lippincott Williams & Wilkins; 2001. p. 465–8 [discussion].
109. Henderson JM. Comment on ref. 77. In: McIntyre FM, editor. Year book of dentistry 2006. Philadelphia: Elsevier Mosby; 2006. p. 173.

Use of Prophylactic Antibiotics in Preventing Infection of Traumatic Injuries

A. Omar Abubaker, DMD, PhD

KEYWORDS

• Prophylactic • Soft tissue • Infection • Trauma

Approximately 11.8 million wounds were treated in the emergency departments in the United States in 2005.[1] At least 7.3 million lacerations are treated annually[2] and an additional 2 million outpatient visits each year occur for treatment of wounds caused by cutting or piercing objects.[3] Half of these traumatic wounds are located on the head and neck,[3,4] This makes it important for clinicians to understand how best to prevent infections following traumatic soft tissue injuries, as well as traumatic bony injuries, in these areas.

The primary goal in the management of traumatic wounds is to achieve rapid healing with optimal functional and esthetic results.[5] This is best accomplished by providing an environment that prevents infection of the wound during healing. Such care includes adequate overall medical assessment of the patient; proper wound evaluation and preparation; adequate anesthesia and hemostasis; reduction of tissue contamination by wound cleansing, debridement of devitalized tissue, and removal of any foreign bodies; and correct wound closure. Several reviews describe the principles and details of this phase of wound care.[6]

Despite good wound care, some infections still occur. Accordingly, some investigators argue that prophylactic antibiotics have an important role in the management of certain types of wounds.[7] This article reviews the basis of antibiotic use in preventing wound infection in general and its use in oral and facial wounds in particular. See the article by Stefanopoulos elsewhere in this issue for a discussion of the role of antibiotics in the management of bite wounds.

A version of this article originally appeared in Abubaker AO. Use of Prophylactic Antibiotics in Preventing Infection of Traumatic Injuries. Oral Max Surg Clin North Am 2009;21:259–64.
Department of Oral and Maxillofacial Surgery, School of Dentistry, Virginia Commonwealth University, Virginia Commonwealth University Medical Center, 521 North 11th Street, PO Box 980566, Richmond, VA 23298, USA
E-mail address: abubaker@vcu.edu

Dent Clin N Am 53 (2009) 707–715
doi:10.1016/j.cden.2009.08.004
0011-8532/09/$ – see front matter © 2009 Elsevier Inc. All rights reserved.

PROPHYLACTIC ANTIBIOTICS IN PATIENTS WITH SKIN WOUNDS

The term *prophylactic antibiotics* implies the use of such antibiotics as a preventive measure in the absence of an established infection.[8,9] Although virtually all traumatic wounds can be considered contaminated with bacteria to some extent, only a small percentage eventually become infected. Accordingly, it is possible that only a subset of high-risk wounds or patients stand to benefit from prophylactic antibiotics.[7] Estimates of the incidence of traumatic wound infection vary widely, depending on the method of study and the population examined, but most studies have found an incidence of 4.5% to 6.3%.[10–13] In a meta-analysis of seven studies, the wound infection rates in the control populations ranged from 1.1% to 12% with a mean of 6%.[14]

When considering the role of antibiotics in preventing wound infection, it is important to consider the risk factors for infection. These factors relate to the nature of the host, the characteristics of the wound, and the treatment used.[15] The host risk factors include extreme young or old age; medical problems, such as diabetes mellitus, chronic renal failure, obesity, malnutrition, and immunocompromising illnesses; and such therapies as corticosteroids and chemotherapeutic agents.[8,9,16,17] Wound factors that increase risk include high bacterial counts in the wound; oil contamination; and crush injury. Risk of infection also varies according to wound depth, configuration, and size.[7,18] Wounds associated with tendons, joints, and bones; puncture wounds; intraoral wounds; and most mammalian wounds are also considered at high risk for infection. Certain treatments, such as the use of epinephrine-containing solutions, may also increase the risk of infection. Furthermore, risk of infection increases with the number of sutures. Finally, risk of infection may be higher with an inexperienced treating doctor than with an experienced one.[19]

When antibiotics are used to prevent infections in traumatic wounds, certain indications are often cited. Such indications include wounds associated with open joints or fractures, human or animal bites, and intraoral lacerations. Despite limited evidence, antibiotics also are recommended for heavily contaminated wounds (eg, those involving soil, feces, saliva, vaginal secretions, or other contaminants).[20] Prophylactic antibiotics also are advocated for traumatic wounds in patients who have prosthetic devices and for preventing bacteremia in patients at risk for developing endocarditis.[20,21] Systemic antibiotics also are recommended when there is a lapse of more than 3 hours since injury, when there is lymphedematous tissue involvement, and when the host is immunocompromised.[22,23]

According to the principles of presurgical prophylaxis, antibiotics, if they are to be given at all, should be administered as soon as possible after the injury, if possible within the first 3 hours, and continued for 3 to 5 days.[7,22,24] The antibiotic therapy should also be directed against the most common skin pathogens, *Staphylococcus aureus* and *Streptococci*.[22] Cloxacillin and first-generation cephalosporins are appropriate as first-line therapy.

Despite the frequent use of prophylactic antibiotics to prevent traumatic wound infections, some clinicians still have reservations about the effectiveness of their use. Some investigators argue that most uncomplicated wounds heal without systemic antibiotic therapy.[22] In addition, in many situations, prophylactic antibiotics not only fail to reduce the overall rate of infection, but also may skew the bacteriology toward more unusual or resistant pathogens.[7] In fact, clinical studies fail to demonstrate a lower infection rate among patients with uncomplicated wounds treated with prophylactic antibiotics than among control subjects,[25] and no randomized trials have shown a clear benefit of antibiotic prophylaxis for simple wounds in immunocompetent patients.[25–30] Furthermore, a meta-analysis of randomized trials found no benefit from the use of prophylactic antibiotics for simple wounds.[24]

Several randomized, controlled studies have examined the ability of antibiotics to prevent infection of simple nonbite wounds managed in the emergency department. A meta-analysis of seven of these studies showed that wound infection rates in the control populations ranged from 1.1% to 12%, with a mean of 6%, with patients treated with antibiotics having a slightly greater risk of infection than untreated controls.[14] More detailed analysis of several subgroups looked at whether or not the wounds were sutured, whether the wounds were located on the hands or elsewhere, what was the route of antibiotic administration (oral vs intramuscular), and what antibiotic type was employed. This analysis also failed to show any benefit for the use of systemic prophylactic antibiotics. In 1995, Cummings and Del Becaro[14] concluded that there was little justification for the routine administration of antibiotics to patients who had simple nonbite wounds managed in the emergency department. However, these investigators were unable to examine the potential benefits of antibiotics in high-risk groups because most of these were excluded from their clinical trials. Accordingly, selection bias remains a problematic issue, with most of the published studies looking at the role of antibiotics in management of traumatic wounds in the emergency department.[15,20]

USE OF PROPHYLACTIC ANTIBIOTICS FOR PREVENTION OF INFECTION OF INTRAORAL WOUNDS

Intraoral wounds, including tongue lacerations and orocutaneous wounds, are commonly encountered in the emergency department. Such wounds can involve the mucosa only or the mucosa and adjacent skin, so-called "through-and-through" lacerations. These wounds are often the result of penetration of the lips by the patient's teeth following minor or major trauma or seizures. Most emergency medicine textbooks consider larger mucosal wounds, particularly those that are through-and-through wounds, to be dirty wounds and at high risk for infection because of the oral bacterial flora. These books generally recommend a course of prophylactic antibiotics to prevent infection after these wounds are repaired.[31,32] Infection has been reported in up to 12% of wounds involving the mucosa only and in up to 33% of through-and-through lacerations[33] Altieri and colleagues[34] studied the benefits of 3 days of penicillin prophylaxis in a randomized, controlled trial of 100 intraoral lacerations managed in a pediatric emergency department. The overall infection rate was found to be 6.4%, with no statistically significant difference between the control (8.5%) and the penicillin (4.4%) groups. Although this study had a limited number of patients enrolled, it concluded that routine antibiotic prophylaxis is unwarranted for simple intraoral lacerations in children, although it may be beneficial in sutured wounds.[35] Steel and colleagues[33] conducted a prospective, randomized, double-blind, controlled study of 5 days of oral penicillin versus placebo therapy in adults. They found a statistically significant difference in the infection rates between compliant patients in the two groups (6.7% for penicillin vs 18.8% in the placebo group). In a subgroup of those patients who had through-and-through lacerations, 7% of the treatment group versus 27% of the control group developed wound infections. These investigators could not conclusively recommend prophylactic penicillin for adults with intraoral lacerations treated within 24 hours after injury. However, the investigators felt that noncompliant patients and those who had through-and-through lacerations may benefit from a course of prophylactic penicillin.[33] Penicillin-allergic patients should receive clindamycin.[15]

Mark and Granquist[35] reviewed the literature on the use of prophylactic oral antibiotics for treatment of intraoral wounds. Only four clinical research articles fulfilled their criteria for inclusion in the review.[33,34,36,37] They concluded that prophylactic oral antibiotics play an inconclusive role in the treatment of intraoral wounds. They also concluded that all published randomized studies to date have failed to demonstrate a statistically significant difference in wound infection rates when antibiotics are compared with placebo or routine wound care. The only placebo-controlled, double-blind, randomized clinical trial evaluating the efficacy of oral prophylactic antibiotic use in simple intraoral wounds had small enrollment numbers and accordingly failed to conclusively demonstrate a statistically significant benefit of such use. Mark and Granquist[35] recommended that until a larger clinical trial is performed, treatment decisions on the use of prophylactic antibiotics for intraoral wounds should be guided by clinical judgment of the practitioner.

The value of antibiotic prophylaxis for lacerations of the tongue is less well studied, although one underpowered study reported no infections in 28 children managed without antibiotics.[38] Accordingly, there is insufficient evidence to make any definitive recommendations with regard to antibiotic prophylaxis for tongue or intraoral lacerations in children.[21]

TOPICAL ANTIBIOTICS FOR TREATMENT OF TRAUMATIC WOUNDS

Application of topical antibiotic ointments has often been proposed to help reduce infection rates and prevent scab formation.[22,25,30,39] Ointments containing bacitracin, neomycin, or polymyxin have been routinely used on simple lacerations by many emergency physicians in the United States.[40] Animal studies have shown that topical antimicrobials inside the wound before closure may reduce the infection rate in contaminated wounds.[41] One double-blind, randomized human trial found a 5% infection rate with antibiotic ointment compared with an unexpectedly high 17.6% rate with a petrolatum jelly control.[42] Other studies, however, have found no significant reduction in infection rates with topical antibiotics.[43] Because of the higher risk of infection with crush injuries when compared with sharp lacerations, some experts recommend topical antibiotics only for stellate wounds with abraded skin edges,[44] but this is not based on comparative trial data. So far, the effectiveness of topical antibiotic ointments in managing minor wounds has not been properly investigated.[7,21] Moreover, despite the frequent use of topical antibiotics, surprisingly few studies have assessed their efficacy after suture wound closure.[7]

ANTIBIOTIC PROPHYLAXIS IN PATIENTS WITH OPEN FRACTURES AND JOINT WOUNDS

Open fracture and joint wounds are a recognizable risk for microbial contamination and subsequent development of osteomyelitis. Any break in the skin (or mucosa) over a fracture that could allow for bacterial access to bone should be considered an open fracture. Open fractures and joint wounds are often classified into three categories according to the mechanism of injury, severity of soft tissue damage, configuration of the fracture, and degree of contamination.[45,46] Type I is an open fracture with a skin wound that is clean and less than 1 cm long; type II is an open fracture with a laceration that is more than 1 cm long, but without evidence of extensive soft tissue damage, flaps, or avulsion; and type III is either an open segmental fracture or an open fracture with extensive soft tissue damage or a traumatic amputation. A prospective, randomized, controlled trial by Patzakis and colleagues[47] on the importance of antibiotics in the treatment of open fractures showed that the infection rates were 13.9%, 10%, and 2.3% in the placebo, penicillin, and cephalosporin groups, respectively. In a follow-up study, Patzakis and Wilkins[48] showed that the single most important factor in reducing the infection rate was early (<3 hours) administration of antibiotics that provide antibacterial activity against both gram-positive and gram-negative organisms.[48] A Cochrane Database review concluded that antibiotics reduce the incidence of infection in open fractures of the limbs when compared with no antibiotics or placebo.[49]

Most investigators agree that the use of antibiotics in the management of open fractures and joint wounds is appropriate. However, the duration of therapy and the optimal antibiotic choices remain unresolved issues.[8] Current recommendations with regard to duration are to continue treatment for 24 hours after wound closure in type I and II injuries and for 72 hours, or for 24 hours after wound closure, in type III injuries.[45,50] For type I and II open fractures, S aureus, Streptococci spp, and aerobic gram-negative bacilli are the most common infecting organisms, and the antibiotic of choice is a first- or second-generation cephalosporin.[45,51] An extended-spectrum quinolone (eg, gatifloxacin or moxifloxacin) is an alternative antibiotic regimen that is currently the preferred choice in the military.[52,53] Type III open fractures may require better coverage for gram-negative organisms by the addition of an aminoglycoside to a cephalosporin.[45] For severe injures with soil or fecal contamination and tissue damage with areas of ischemia, it is recommended that penicillin be added to provide coverage against anaerobes, particularly Clostridia spp.[8] Antibiotic coverage for other bacteria may also be needed for certain environmental exposures, such as farm accidents (Clostridium), combat casualty wounds (Acinetobacter, Pseudomonas, Clostridium), fresh water exposure (Aeromonas, Pseudomonas), and salt water exposure (Aeromonas, Vibrio).[51,54]

Antibiotic therapy for prophylactic management of open fractures resulting from gunshot wounds warrants special consideration and depends in part on whether the injury was caused by a low- or high-velocity missile.[8] In fractures associated with low-velocity wounds treated with a closed technique, the infection rate with antibiotic prophylaxis is about the same as the infection rate without antibiotic prophylaxis (3% in both groups).[55] However, wounds caused by high-velocity gunshot injuries are associated with increased risk of infection, and antibiotic therapy is generally recommended for 48 to 72 hours.[56] Although a first-generation cephalosporin with or without an aminoglycoside is recommended for most patients, penicillin should be added to provide additional anaerobic coverage of Clostridia spp in grossly contaminated wounds.[57] The Eastern Surgical Society for the Surgery of Trauma has developed treatment guidelines for use of prophylactic antibiotics in open fractures. For type I and type II fractures, these guidelines recommend antibiotic therapy directed against gram-positive bacteria (first-generation cephalosporins) be administered within 6 hours of the injury and for 24 hours after wound closure. For type III fractures, antibiotic therapy should be directed against gram-positive and gram-negative bacteria, be given within 6 hours following the fracture, and be continued for 72 hours, or for 24 hours after wound closure.[45]

In the oral and maxillofacial region, guidelines in the literature are less clear-cut about the use of prophylactic antibiotic to prevent infection when soft tissue injury is associated with facial fractures. A systematic review revealed four randomized studies that examined the possible benefit of prophylactic antibiotics in such situations.[58] This review included studies related to facial factures with and without facial skin or mucosal lacerations.[59-63] The investigators concluded that only compound fractures of the body and angle of the mandible would benefit from a short-term course of prophylactic antibiotics (<48 hours). The review did not address the relationship between soft tissue lacerations, facial fractures, and the use of prophylactic antibiotics, although the investigators suggested that the benefit of prophylactic antibiotics is likely to be related to their effect on bacterial contamination from the dentition and through the periodontal ligament.[58]

SUMMARY

The wide use, misuse, and overuse of prophylactic antibiotics likely contribute significantly to overall health care cost. One of the areas of potential misuse of these agents is in the prevention of infection of traumatic wounds. This review shows that despite the widespread use of prophylactic antibiotics to prevent infection of wound injuries, the scientific data to support such wide use are limited to specific situations and for limited periods of time. These situations include those involving immunocompromised patients; grossly contaminated wounds; delayed wound closure; patients at high risk for endocarditis; patients with open fractures and joint wounds; and high-velocity gunshot wounds. There may also be a benefit of such use for short duration when facial or oral lacerations are associated with compound fractures of the mandible and in through-and-through lacerations of the mouth in adults. There appears to be no benefit for prophylactic antibiotics for simple facial skin lacerations, tongue lacerations, and intraoral lacerations when they are not associated with facial fractures.

REFERENCES

1. Nawar EW, Niska RW, Xu J. National Hospital Ambulatory Medical Care Survey: 2005 emergency department summary. Advance data from vital health statistics. No. 386. Hyattsville (MD): National Center for Health Statistics; 2007.
2. Singer AJ, Thode HC, Hollander JE. National trends in ED lacerations between 1992 and 2002. Am J Emerg Med 2006;24:183–8.
3. Hing E, Cherry DK, Woodwell DA. National Ambulatory Medical Care Survey: 2004 summary. Advance data from vital and health statistics. No. 374. Hyattsville (MD): National Center for Health Statistics; 2006.
4. Hollander GE, Singer JA. State of the art laceration management. Ann Emerg Med 1999;34:356–67.
5. Singer AJ, Dagum AB. Current management of acute cutaneous wounds. N Engl J Med 2008;359:1037–46.
6. Capellan O, Hollander JE. Management of lacerations in the emergency department. Emerg Med Clin North Am 2003;21:205–31.
7. Moran GJ, Talan DA, Abrahamian FD. Antimicrobial prophylaxis for wounds and procedures in the emergency department. Infect Dis Clin North Am 2008;22: 117–43.
8. Holtom PD. Antibiotic prophylaxis: current recommendations. J Am Acad Orthop Surg 2006;14:S98–100.
9. Mangram AJ, Horan TC, Pearson ML, et al. Guideline for prevention of surgical site infection. 1999; Hospital Infection Control Practices Advisory Committee. Infect Control Hosp Epidemiol 1999;20:250–78.
10. Gosnold JK. Infection rate of sutured wounds. Practitioner 1977;218:584–5.
11. Hutton PA, Jones BM, Law DJ. Depot penicillin as prophylaxis in accidental wounds. Br J Surg 1978;65:549–50.
12. Rutherford WH, Spence R. Infection in wounds sutured in the accident and emergency department. Ann Emerg Med 1980;9:350–2.
13. Thirlby RC, Blair AJ, Thal ER. The value of prophylactic antibiotics for simple lacerations. Surg Gynecol Obstet 1983;156:212–6.
14. Cummings P, Del Beccaro MA. Antibiotics to prevent infection of simple wounds: a meta-analysis of randomized studies. Am J Emerg Med 1995;13:396–400.
15. Nakamura Y, Daya M. Use of appropriate antimicrobials in wound management. Emerg Med Clin North Am 2007;25:159–76.

16. Singer AJ, Hollander JE, Quinn JV. Evaluation and management of traumatic lacerations. N Engl J Med 1997;337:1142–8.
17. Cruse PJE, Foord R. A five-year prospective study of 23,469 surgical wounds. Arch Surg 1973;107:206–9.
18. Hollander JE, Singer AJ, Valantine SM, et al. Risk infection in patients with traumatic laceration. Acad Emerg Med 2001;8:716–20.
19. Lammers RL, Hudson DL, Seaman ME. Prediction of traumatic wound infection with a neural network-derived decision model. Am J Emerg Med 2003;21:1–7.
20. Wedmore IS. Wound care: modern evidence in the treatment of man's age-old injuries. Emerg Med Pract 2005;7:1–24.
21. Goulin S, Patel H. Office management of minor wounds. Can Fam Physician 2001;47:769–74.
22. Eron LJ. Targeting lurking pathogens in acute traumatic and chronic wounds. J Emerg Med 1999;17:189–95.
23. Horetg FM, King C. Textbook of pediatric emergency procedures. Baltimore (MD): Williams & Wilkins; 1997. Chap 7, p. 43–9; Chap1101, p. 125–39.
24. Gravett A, Sterner S, Clinton JE, et al. A trial of povidone-iodine in the prevention of infection in sutured lacerations. Ann Emerg Med 1987;16:167–71.
25. Barkin RM, Caputo GL, Jaffe DM, et al. Pediatric emergency medicine, concepts and clinical practice. 2nd edition. St Louis (MO): Mosby; 1997. Chap 32, p. 439–75.
26. Quinn JV, Wells G, Sutcliffe T, et al. Tissue adhesive versus suture wound repair at 1 year: randomized clinical trial correlating early, 3-month, and 1-year cosmetic outcome. Ann Emerg Med 1998;32:645–9.
27. Singer AJ, Hollander JB, Valantine SM, et al. Prospective, randomized, controlled trials of tissue adhesive 2-octycyanoacrylate vs standard wound closure techniques for laceration repair. Acad Emerg Med 1998;5:94–9.
28. Bruns TB, Simon Hk, McLario DJ, et al. Laceration repair using a tissue adhesive in a children's emergency department. Pediatrics 1996;98:673–5.
29. Quinn JV, Drzewiecki A, Li MM, et al. A randomized, controlled trial comparing a tissue adhesive with suturing in the repair of pediatric facial lacerations. Ann Emerg Med 1993;22:23–7.
30. Kunisad T, Yamada K, Oda S, et al. Investigation on the efficacy of povidone-iodine against antiseptic-resistant species. Dermatology 1997;195(Suppl 2):14–8.
31. Tintinalli JE, Kelen GD, Stapczynski JS, editors. Emergency medicine: a comprehensive study guide. 6th edition. New York: McGraw-Hill; 2004.
32. Marx JA, Hockberger RS, Walls RM, editors. Marx: Rosen's emergency medicine: concepts and clinical practice. 6th edition. Philadelphia: Mosby Elsevier; 2006.
33. Steel MT, Sainsbury CR, Robinson WA, et al. Prophylactic penicillin for intraoral wounds. Ann Emerg Med 1989;18:847–52.
34. Altieri M, Brasch L, Getson P. Antibiotic prophylaxis in intraoral wounds. Am J Emerg Med 1986;4:507–10.
35. Mark DJ, Granquist EJ. Are prophylactic oral antibiotics indicated for the treatment of intraoral wounds? Ann Emerg Med 2008;52:368–72.
36. Goldberg MH. Antibiotics and oral and oral-cutaneous lacerations. J Oral Surg 1965;23:117–22.
37. Paterson JA, Cardo VA Jr, Stratigos GT. An examination of antibiotic prophylaxis in oral and maxillofacial surgery. J Oral Surg 1970;28:753–9.
38. Lamell CW, Fraone G, Casamassimo MS, et al. Presenting characteristics and treatment outcomes for tongue lacerations in children. Pediatr Dent 1999;21:34–8.

39. Bikowski J. Secondarily infected wounds and dermatoses: a diagnosis and treatment guide. J Emerg Med 1999;17:197–206.
40. Howell JM, Chisholm CD. Outpatient wound preparation and care: a national survey. Ann Emerg Med 1992;24:976–81.
41. Edlich RF, Smith QT, Edgerton MT. Resistance of the surgical wound to antimicrobial prophylaxis and its mechanisms of development. Am J Surg 1973;126: 583–91.
42. Dire DJ, Coppola M, Dwyer DA, et al. A prospective evaluation of topical antibiotics for preventing infections in uncomplicated soft-tissue wounds repaired in the ED. Acad Emerg Med 1995;2:4–10.
43. Caro D, Reynolds KW. An investigation to evaluate a topical antibiotic in the prevention of wound sepsis in a casualty department. Br J Clin Pract 1967;21: 605–7.
44. Edlich RF, Sutton ST. Post repair wound care revisited. Acad Emerg Med 1995;2: 2–3.
45. Luchette FA, Bone LB, Born CT, et al. East Practice Management Guidelines Work Group: practice management guidelines for prophylactic antibiotic use in open fractures. Available at: http://www.east.org/. Accessed November 18, 2006.
46. Gustilo RB, Mendoza RM, Williams DN. Problems in the management of type III (severe) open fractures. A new classification of type III open fractures. J Trauma 1984;24:742–6.
47. Patzakis MJ, Harvey JP Jr, Ivler D. The role of antibiotics in the management of open fractures. J Bone Joint Surg Am 1974;56:532–41.
48. Patzakis MJ, Wilkins J. Factors influencing infection rate in open fracture wounds. Clin Orthop Relat Res 1989;243:36–40.
49. Gosselin RI, Roberts I, Gillespie WJ. Antibiotics for preventing infection in open limb fractures. Cochrane Database Syst Rev 2004;(1):CD003764.
50. Calhoun J, Sexton DJ, et al. Adult posttraumatic osteomyelitis. Up to Date 2006; ver 14.3. Available at: www.uptodate.com. Acccessed November 16, 2008.
51. Templeman DC, Gulli B, Tsukayama DT, et al. Update on the management of open fractures of the tibial shaft. Clin Orthop Relat Res 1998;350:18–25.
52. Patzakis MJ, Banis RS, Lee J, et al. Prospective randomized, double-blind study comparing agent antibiotic therapy, ciprofloxacin, to combination antibiotic therapy in open fracture wounds. J Orthop Trauma 2000;14:529–33.
53. Butler F. Antibiotics in facial combat casualty care 2002. Mil Med 2003;168: 911–4.
54. Davis SC, Cazzaniga AL, Eaglstein WH, et al. Over-the-counter topical antimicrobials: effective treatments? Arch Dermatol Res 2005;297:190–5.
55. Dickey RL, Barnes BC, Kearns RJ, et al. Efficacy of antibiotics in low-velocity gunshot fractures. J Orthop Trauma 1989;3:6–10.
56. Heenessy MJ, Banks HH, Leach RB. Extremity gunshot wound and gunshot fracture in civilian practice. Clin Orthop Relat Res 1976;114:296–303.
57. Simpson BM, Wilson RH, Grant RE. Antibiotic therapy in gunshot wound injuries. Clin Orthop Relat Res 2003;408:82–5.
58. Anderasen JO, Jensen S, Schwartz O, et al. A systemic review of prophylactic antibiotics in the surgical treatment of maxillofacial fractures. J Oral Maxillofac Surg 2006;64:1664–8.
59. Chole RA, Yee J. Antibiotic prophylaxis for facial fractures. Arch Otolaryngol Head Neck Surg 1987;113:1055–7.
60. Zallen RD, Curry JT. A study of antibiotic usage in compound mandibular fractures. J Oral Surg 1975;33:431–4.

61. Aderhold L, Jung H, Frenkel G. Untersuchungen űber den wert einer Antibiotika Prophylaxe bei kiefer-Gesichtsverletzungen-eine prospective studie. Dtsch Zahnärztl Z 1983;38:402–7.
62. Gerlach KL, Pape HD. Untersuchungen zur Antibiotikaprophylaxe bei der operativen Behandlung von Unterkieferfrakturen. Dtsch Z Mund Kiefer Gesichtschir 1988;12:497–502.
63. Abubaker AO, Rollert MK. Postoperative antibiotic prophylaxis in mandibular fractures: a preliminary randomized, double-blind, and placebo-controlled clinical study. J Oral Maxillofac Surg 2001;59:1415–9.

Cone Beam CT for Diagnosis and Treatment Planning in Trauma Cases

Leena Palomo, DDS, MSD[a], J. Martin Palomo, DDS, MSD[b,c],*

KEYWORDS

• Cone beam computed tomography
• Three dimensional imaging • Trauma • Technology

Three-dimensional imaging offers many advantages in making diagnoses and planning treatment. This article focuses on cone beam CT (CBCT) for making diagnoses and planning treatment in trauma-related cases. CBCT equipment is smaller and less expensive than traditional medical CT equipment and is tailored to address challenges specific to the dentoalveolar environment. Like medical CT, CBCT offers a three-dimensional view that conventional two-dimensional dental radiography fails to provide. CBCT combines the strengths of medical CT with those of conventional dental radiography to accommodate unique diagnostic and treatment-planning applications that have particular utility in dentoalveolar trauma cases. CBCT is useful, for example, in identifying tooth fractures relative to surrounding alveolar bone, in determining alveolar fracture location and morphology, in analyzing ridge-defect height and width, and in imaging temporomandibular joints. Treatment-planning applications include those involving extraction of fractured teeth, placement of implants, exposure of impacted teeth, and analyses of airways.

In hospital settings, it is common to use CT in patients with trauma and pathologic conditions. However, in dental practice, practitioners depend almost entirely on two-dimensional plain films. The applications and advantages of the third dimension in dental medicine still remain largely unrealized.

---

[a] Department of Periodontics, Case School of Dental Medicine, Case Western Reserve University, 10900 Euclid Avenue, Cleveland, OH 44106, USA
[b] Department of Orthodontics, Case School of Dental Medicine, 10900 Euclid Avenue, Cleveland, OH 44106, USA
[c] Craniofacial Imaging Center, Case School of Dental Medicine, Case Western Reserve University, 10900 Euclid Avenue, Cleveland, OH 44106, USA
* Corresponding author. Department of Orthodontics, Case School of Dental Medicine, 10900 Euclid Avenue, Cleveland, OH 44106.
E-mail address: palomo@case.edu (J.M. Palomo).

Dent Clin N Am 53 (2009) 717–727
doi:10.1016/j.cden.2009.07.001
0011-8532/09/$ – see front matter © 2009 Elsevier Inc. All rights reserved.

In 1998, Mozzo and colleagues[1] reported on the NewTom 9000 (Quantitative Radiology, Verona, Italy), the first CBCT unit developed specifically for dental use. Other similar devices introduced at around that time included the Ortho-CT, which was renamed the 3DX (J. Morita Mfg. Corp., Kyoto, Japan) multi-image micro-CT in 2000.[2] In 2003, Hashimoto and colleagues[3] reported that the 3DX CBCT produced better image quality with a much lower radiation dose than the then newest multidetector row helical CT unit (1.19 mSv versus 458 mSv per examination).

Two major differences distinguish CBCT machines from conventional hospital CT scanners (helical, spiral, fan). First, CBCT uses a low-energy fixed anode tube, similar to that used in dental panoramic radiograph machines. Second, CBCT machines rotate around the patient only once, capturing the data using a cone-shaped x-ray beam. These differences make possible a less-expensive, smaller machine that exposes the patient to approximately 20% of the radiation of a helical CT, which is equivalent to a typical exposure from a full-mouth periapical series.[4,5] The volumetric capturing difference provides CBCT with a more focused beam, resulting in images with higher geometric accuracy, higher spatial resolution, and considerably less scattering in comparison with images from conventional CT scanners. One disadvantage of the volumetric capturing method is that the Hounsfield units, which provide density information, cannot currently be captured in a reliable fashion when using CBCT. Ongoing projects are working on such calibration, but no method is currently commercially available.

Due to CBCT's volumetric data capturing method, related articles have referred to this technology with a variety of terms including cone beam volumetric tomography, cone beam computed volumetric tomography, cone beam volumetric radiography, dental CT, dental volume tomography, digital volumetric tomography, and cone beam 3D. This multiplicity of terms stems largely from disagreement over whether CBCT capturing methods can truly be called tomography. The result is a lack of terminology consensus in the literature, making it more difficult for researchers and clinicians to stay up to date with the latest projects and publications because different key words need to be searched.

All of the CBCT scanners on the market use the same volumetric capturing technology, but have significant hardware differences. Scanners can be categorized according to type of detector, patient position (sitting, standing, or supine), field of view, the use of fixed radiation settings or user-controlled settings, and whether or not the scanner is dedicated or hybrid. The detector can be either an amorphous silicon flat-panel detector or a combination of an image intensifier and a charge-coupled device camera. Both these technologies have been proven to be accurate and reliable and provide sufficient resolution for dental medicine needs. The field of view stands for the final image size produced by the scanner. Different scanners offer different field-of-view capabilities resulting in images ranging in size from 1 in to 12 in. To best accommodate collimation capabilities and reduced radiation exposure as much as possible, the field of view used should match the region of interest. In other words, if all the clinician wants is to evaluate an area of suspected fracture, the relationship of the alveolar ridge to an impacted tooth, or area of suspected pathology, there is no need to capture an image that would show the patient's entire head. Some scanners offer both large and small field-of-view capabilities, while others, tailored for more specific applications, offer only small field-of-view capabilities.

A significant lack of standardization found in the commercially available CBCT scanners has to do with the radiological settings. Depending on the scanner, the milliamperage used may range from 1 mA to 15 mA, with most scanners using around 6 mA. Often the radiological settings are fixed and cannot be changed without the intervention of the manufacturer's engineers. So radiation exposure depends largely on the scanner used, since it plays an important role on the settings used.

Effective CBCT radiation dose depends on the settings used (kilovolt [peak] and milliampere), collimation, and exposure time. The use of lower settings reduces the radiation dose received by the patient, but could also diminish image quality.[6] The choice should always be the lowest possible settings that also accommodate a diagnostic-quality image. However, specific settings for different clinical applications have yet to be determined. This can only be done by considering the image quality because radiation exposure information without image quality control is just half the story.[7] The settings, including milliampere, kilovolt (peak), and field of view, are going to be different for different clinical applications. For example, as the settings for diagnostic screening will differ from those for implant planning. Settings should be consistent among imaging centers, and the scanners should have such settings as options. This is the only way to efficiently apply the ALARA (as low as reasonably achievable) principle.

Within every field, the introduction of new technology raises several fundamental questions, such as: For what practical applications can the new technology be used? and: Is the new technology truly superior to existing modalities? These questions are not easily answered, but require research and comparison. CBCT diagnostics in posttraumatic clinical applications appear to offer advantages over medical CT and conventional dental radiography.

Because all images can be taken in around 10 seconds with a single rotation of the x-ray source, CBCT is useful in trauma, intraoperative, and sedation cases.

CLINICAL APPLICATIONS IN TRAUMA DIAGNOSIS: OVERCOMING CONVENTIONAL CT DIAGNOSTIC CHALLENGES AND ADDING A NEW DIMENSION TO CONVENTIONAL RADIOGRAPHY

CBCT equipment is smaller and less expensive than medical CT equipment and is particularly well suited to evaluating the jaws because of a lower level of metal artifacts in reconstructions versus its helical predecessor. In a conventional CT, for instance, an area of the jaws close to a metallic restoration, a crown, or an implant is difficult to analyze because of the artifacts and distortions that the metal in the region of interest creates. On a CBCT image, the area around metal is usually of diagnostic quality, and with little scattering and no distortion (**Fig. 1**). When compared with dental panoramic radiograph, CBCT is useful in identifying the location of cortical plate fracture that is not through and through (**Fig. 2**). Additionally, CBCT is more sensitive and accurate in imaging the maxilla and mandible. It is reported that mandibular fractures not evident in conventional CT can be identified using CBCT. Also, when using CBCT, as compared to CT and conventional radiograph, information about dentoalveolar fractures is more detailed.[8] This makes CBCT uniquely useful in alveolar fracture diagnosis.

Another common diagnostic challenge is presurgical evaluation of mandibular lingual cortical bone. During open reduction of mandibular fractures, not all fracture sites can be readily exposed for direct visualization.[9] CBCT allows for fracture diagnosis. Similarly, the lingual cortical plate, although not fractured through and through, may present with a concavity or alveolar bone defect. This concavity or defect complicates dental-implant placement either by appearing to have wider alveolar ridge than what is actually there, or by limiting the amount of space available between bone and the inferior alveolar canal. Visualization of alveolar bone morphology and the relationship to other structures, such as the inferior alveolar canal, can be clearly identified using CBCT (**Fig. 3**).

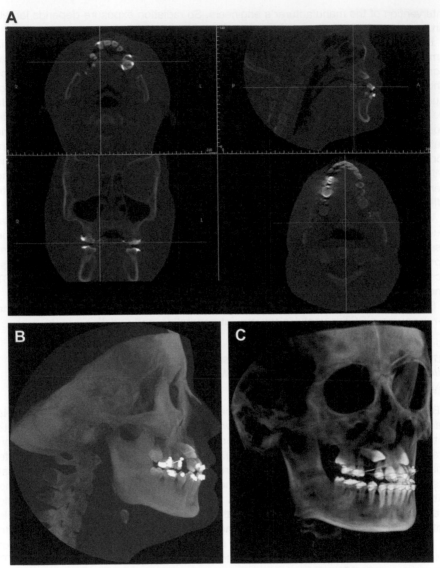

Fig. 1. CBCT images show less scattering and no distortions next to metallic restorations. (*A*) Axial, sagittal, and coronal views of patient with bands and braces. (*B*) Maximum intensity projection view of patient wearing braces and an orthodontic arch wire. (*C*) Volume rendering of same patient, showing how the metal in the area shows no distortion or interference with diagnostic quality.

Location of alveolar ridge relative to anatomic structures, such as the inferior alveolar nerve, maxillary sinus, mental foramen, and adjacent teeth, are readily identified using CBCT. The CBCT image allows for precise measurement of the ridge area and volume in relation to local anatomy (**Fig. 4**) and thus increases diagnostic confidence.

Furthermore, three-dimensional imaging captures skeletal and soft tissue details. Both can be displayed together to examine the relationship of fracture to soft tissue (**Fig. 5**) or individually to examine the details of either. The resulting images are

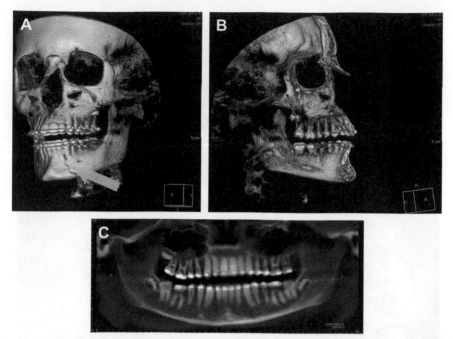

Fig. 2. CBCT image of a 13-year-old male patient. (*A*) Facial view shows buccal cortical plate fracture (*arrow*). (*B*) Lingual view shows no fracture to lingual plate. (*C*) Fracture is visible on panoramic radiograph, with no distinction possible if the fracture is buccal, lingual, or both.

user-friendly, provide far more information than conventional two-dimensional radiographs, and lack the inherent distortion found in conventional radiography. All possible two-dimensional views taken with conventional radiography can be created from a single CBCT scan, which can take less than 10 seconds. One possible reconstruction is the conventional dental panoramic image (**Fig. 6**). A single CBCT following a traumatic event quickly captures a significant amount of useful patient information for diagnosis.

IMPLANT PLANNING

Implantologists have long appreciated the usefulness of three-dimensional imaging, especially for handling posttrauma restoration cases. In the case of trauma, multiple

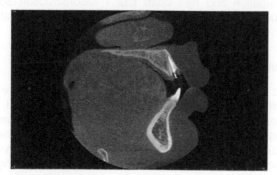

Fig. 3. Twelve-year-old male patient with anterior facial trauma. CBCT reconstruction shows #9 tooth fracture, thinner than 2 mm, but intact buccal plate, and the bucco-lingual relationship of the fractured root to the alveolar ridge.

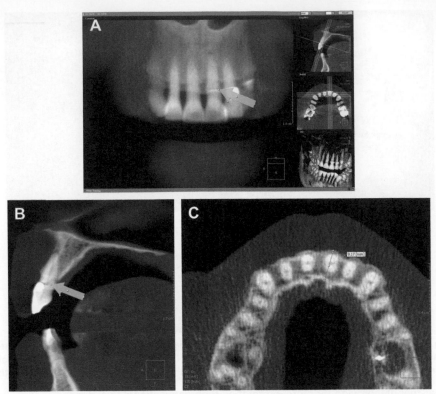

Fig. 4. Seventy-four–year-old male patient with anterior facial trauma. (*A*) CBCT reconstruction shows evidence of #9 root surface fracture (*arrow*). (*B*) Sagittal view confirms fracture of #9 root surface (*arrow*) with no evidence of alveolar fracture. This view also allows for measurement of buccal cortical plate thickness and location of fractured root in the alveolus. (*C*) Measurement tool enables precise measurement of buccolingual ridge thickness.

implants are often necessary. CBCT images, unlike conventional dental radiography, clearly identify buccolingual alveolar ridge deficiency. Conventional CT scans have been used to assess the osseous dimensions, relative bone density, cortical plate thickness, and alveolar ridge height. CBCT technology makes this information available with less radiation and less cost. CBCT reconstruction software includes measurement tools that can be used to measure height, cortical thickness, and distance between landmarks (**Fig. 7**).

CONE BEAM CT–GUIDED IMPLANT PLACEMENT SURGERY

Once the trauma patient is stabilized, the fractured alveolar bone and debris are removed, the soft tissue and mucogingival surgery is completed, and preimplant bone grafting is completed and healed, the case is ready for implant restoration phase. Mounted diagnostic cases and photographs are prepared for diagnostic work-up. A CBCT scan appliance is made with radiopaque pins for barium teeth. A CBCT is taken using settings appropriate to specific products being used. Setting protocols vary depending on the CBCT scanner used. Also, settings of surgical guide software may vary. These specific settings should be verified before scanning. Once scanned, the image is analyzed. Virtual planning involves identifying adequate diameter, length,

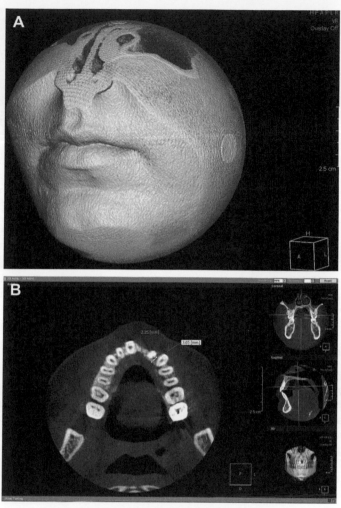

Fig. 5. Twenty-two-year-old female patient with anterior facial trauma, #9 avulsion, and #10 luxation. (*A*) CBCT shows facial soft tissue. (*B*) CBCT shows buccolingual width of postavulsion defect, #9 edentulous area, and #10 luxation area.

and number of implants. Many planning software products accommodate selection of brand-name implants and allow for selection of placement location and angulation such that available bone is used and local anatomy, such as adjacent teeth, nerves, and sinuses, are avoided. Even the bone quality can be somewhat assessed when virtually placing the implants (**Fig. 8**). In the case of trauma, it is important to avoid other traumatized areas where bone grafting was not completed. Bone to house the selected implants at those particular positions is verified directly on top of the CBCT image. Laboratory-fabricated stereolithographic guides are useful for transferring the planned surgery to the patient. This way, virtually planned locations and angulations can be accurately and predictably re-created in patients during surgery. In cases lacking adequate anchorage for surgical guide stability during surgery, such as in cases with multiple missing teeth along with alveolar, trabecular fractures, such products as anchorage pins are useful.

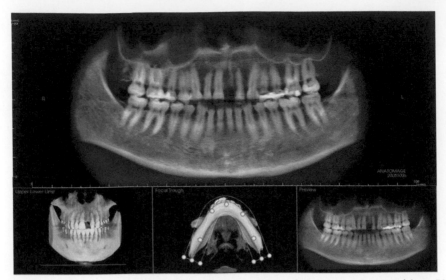

Fig. 6. Twenty-two-year-old female patient with anterior facial trauma, #9 avulsion, #10 luxation. Panoramic reconstruction available based on CBCT data. Note panoramic reconstruction does not give information about bucco-lingual ridge width. CBCT axial slice data in **Fig. 5** reveals bucco-lingual ridge width defect.

AIRWAY ANALYSIS: AN ANCILLARY BENEFIT

CBCT can be used as an improved method for evaluating airways (**Fig. 9**). Conventionally, airway analysis has been done using lateral cephalograms. A comparison of lateral cephalograms to CBCT shows a moderate variation in the measurement of the upper airway area and volume.[10] CBCT has also demonstrated significant differences in measurements of airway volume and the anterioposterior dimension of the oropharyngeal airway between obstructive sleep apnea patients and gender-matched control.[11] Three-dimensional airway analysis is useful when sedation is planned for dental reconstruction. Preliminary studies show that three-dimensional image

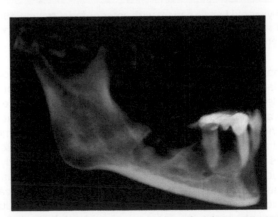

Fig. 7. Forty-seven-year-old female patient with blunt facial trauma, avulsion #30. Buccal cortical fracture, avulsed tooth, and close proximity of defect to inferior alveolar canal are apparent. Additionally, measurement tools are available for precise measurement.

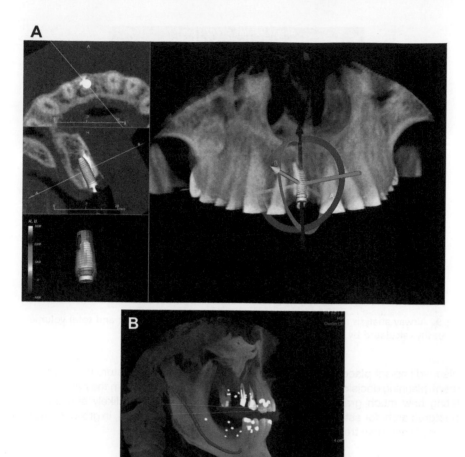

Fig. 8. (*A*) By using density differences, not only is bone quality apparent, but so also are anatomic landmarks that lend themselves to density changes, such as the inferior alveolar canal. Surgical stents for the placement of dental implants can be made using radiopaque markers, to avoid local anatomy. (*B*) Bone quality can be assessed based on density values collected during scanning. The different density values can be displayed with different colors for easy visualization.

reconstructions are useful as "virtual laryngoscopy" in airway management during general anesthesia.[12]

Because trauma cases, once stabilized, are transferred to the operating room for surgical correction, an ancillary benefit of the CBCT originally taken for diagnostics, is the usefulness in anesthesia planning. Additional research and protocol development are needed for this application.

BONE GRAFT ANALYSIS

Volumetric analysis offers better prediction of defect morphology. Understanding the morphology of a traumatic defect is critical in developing the implant site before

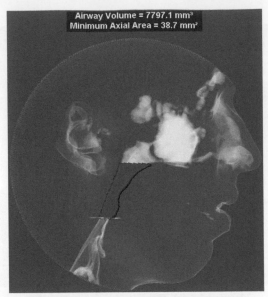

Airway Volume = 7797.1 mm³
Minimum Axial Area = 38.7 mm²

Fig. 9. Airway analysis using CBCT. The area of maximum constriction and total volume can be easily calculated by using automatic segmentation.

planned implant placement. Defect size and shape affect the factors that guide treatment-planning decisions. For example, defect size and shape form the basis for calculating how much graft material is needed, for predicting the likely stability of the postgraft arch, for estimating quality of bone graft over time, and, in growing patients, for predicting how treatment will affect overall facial growth.[13]

SUMMARY

Trauma cases present with a wide range of diagnostic challenges. Not all of these are addressed by either medical CT or conventional dental radiography alone. By comparison, CBCT by itself can often deliver enough information for a diagnosis in one quick scan. It is useful in identification of fracture and defect morphology. It is also useful for determining defect dimensions and the relative locations of pertinent anatomic structures. Such information is needed for planning restorations that involve alveolar bone augmentation and implant placement. Additionally, CBCT shows promise in airway identification, an application that can be developed to reduce operating room occupation times. CBCT in posttraumatic applications enables dentists to address many patient needs.

REFERENCES

1. Mozzo P, Procacci C, Tacconi A, et al. A new volumetric CT machine for dental imaging based on the cone-beam technique: preliminary results. Eur Radiol 1998;8(9):1558–64.
2. Arai Y, Tammisalo E, Iwai K, et al. Development of a compact computed tomographic apparatus for dental use. Dentomaxillofac Radiol 1999;28:245–8.
3. Hashimoto K, Yoshinori A, Kazui I, et al. A comparison of a new, limited cone beam computed tomography machine for dental use with a multidetector row

helical CT machine. Oral Surg Oral Med Oral Pathol Oral Radiol Endod 2003;95: 371–7.

4. Mah JK, Danforth RA, Bumann A, et al. Radiation absorbed in maxillofacial imaging with a new dental computed tomography device. Oral Surg Oral Med Oral Pathol Oral Radiol Endod 2003;96:508–13.

5. Schulze D, Heiland M, Thurmann H, et al. Radiation exposure during midfacial imaging using 4- and 16-slice computed tomography, cone beam computed tomography systems and conventional radiography. Dentomaxillofac Radiol 2004;33:83–6.

6. Palomo JM, Rao PS, Hans MG. Influence of CBCT exposure conditions on radiation dose. Oral Surg Oral Med Oral Pathol Oral Radiol Endod 2008;105(6): 773–82.

7. Ballrick J, Palomo JM, Ruch E, et al. Resolution of a commercially available CBCT. Am J Orthod Dentofacial Orthop 2008;134(4):573–82.

8. Ilgüy D, Ilgüy M, Fisekcioglu E, et al. Detection of jaw and root fractures using cone beam computed tomography: a case report. Dentomaxillofac Radiol 2009;38(3):169–73.

9. Pohlenz P, Blessmann M, Blake F, et al. Major mandibular surgical procedures as an indication for intraoperative imaging. J Oral Maxillofac Surg 2008;66(2):324–9.

10. Aboudara CA, Hatcher D, Nielsen IL, et al. A three-dimensional evaluation of the upper airway in adolescents. Orthod Craniofac Res 2003;6(Suppl 1):173–5.

11. Ogawa T, Enciso R, Memon A. Evaluation of 3D airway imaging of obstructive sleep apnea with cone-beam computed tomography. Stud Health Technol Inform 2005;111:365–8.

12. Osorio F, Perilla M, Doyle DJ, et al. Cone beam computed tomography: an innovative tool for airway assessment. Anesth Analg 2008;106(6):1803–7.

13. Quereshy FA, Savell TA, Palomo JM. Applications of cone beam CT in the practice of oral and maxillofacial surgery. J Oral Maxillofac Surg 2008;66(4):791–6.

Preventive Strategies for Traumatic Dental Injuries

Cecilia Bourguignon[a,b,]*, Asgeir Sigurdsson[b,c,d,e]

KEYWORDS

- Dental injuries • Prevention • Education
- Preventive appliances • Mouthguards • Sports

Traumatic dental and maxillofacial injuries are common occurrences, and affect worldwide approximately 20% to 30% of the permanent dentition, often with serious esthetic, functional, psychological, and economic consequences. With such a high frequency of injuries, prevention becomes a primary goal. A prevention approach relies on the identification of etiologic factors, and on giving rise to measures aimed at avoiding those factors or at reducing their impact (**Fig. 1**).

Several epidemiologic studies have examined the etiology of injuries. However, only a few have offered analysis leading to indications of preventive measures that could be instituted to interfere in the etiology of injuries.[1–3] **Fig. 1** shows data regarding the environment in which the traumatic injuries occur: traffic, home, school, and others. It appears from **Fig. 1** that injuries in those older than 7 years occur more frequently during sports activities. Fortunately, sport is the activity for which preventive measures seem feasible and that may be effective in reducing the rate and severity of oral trauma. Traffic accidents are the next most frequent cause of oral trauma, and here also preventive measures to avoid or reduce the consequences of severe impacts are feasible.

A significant number of oral and dental injuries result from contact sports such as American football, basketball, rugby, soccer, boxing, wrestling, or "stick sports" (**Fig. 2**). However, there is a growing indication that oral and dental injuries occur as much if not more often during children's play or leisure activities.[1,2] For example, in a study by Skaare and Jacobsen[2] in Norway in 2003, nearly half (48%) of the 1275 injured individuals reported were injured at school. Sports and traffic accidents were less common in their sample. Organized sports accidents represented only

[a] Endodontics and Dental Traumatology Clinic, 6 Rue Benouville, 75 116 Paris, France
[b] International Association of Dental Traumatology
[c] University of North Carolina School of Dentistry, Chapel Hill, North Carolina, USA
[d] UCL Eastman Dental Institute, London, United Kingdom
[e] Holan ehf, Hatun 2a, 105 Reykjavik, Iceland
* Corresponding author. Endodontics and Dental Traumatology, 6 Rue Benouville, 75 116 Paris, France.
E-mail address: cecilia.bourguignon@libertysurf.fr (C. Bourguignon).

Dent Clin N Am 53 (2009) 729–749
doi:10.1016/j.cden.2009.06.002
0011-8532/09/$ – see front matter © 2009 Published by Elsevier Inc.

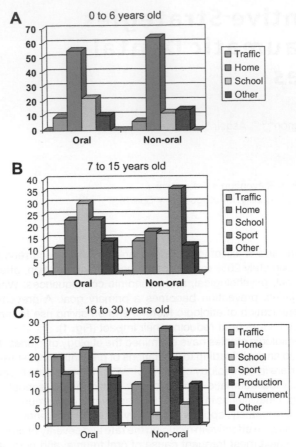

Fig. 1. (*A–C*) Injury environment for oral and nonoral injuries at various ages. An epidemiologic study on injuries during 1 year in a Swedish county. (*Data from* Peterson EE, Andersson L, Sörensen S. Traumatic oral versus non-oral injuries. An epidemilogical study during 1 year in a Swedish county. Swed Dent J 1997;21(1–2):55–68.)

8% of the total number of injuries, similar to the number of individuals injured by violence. The investigators concluded that probably only one-third of the injuries were preventable. The same results were reported by Andreasen[3] in 2001 from a sample of 3655 dental casualty insurance claims from a major Danish insurance company. Thus, 7% of the dental trauma claims were due to organized sports whereas 93% resulted from varied and unpreventable causes. In both studies, the investigators felt that it is neither easy to prevent dental injuries nor to create guidelines on prevention. Based on these studies, it seems that promoting the use of mouthguards and facial masks is an insufficient strategic measure to prevent oral trauma.

EDUCATION AS A PREVENTIVE STRATEGY FOR TRAUMATIC DENTAL INJURIES

The best strategic measure for preventing dental and oral injuries is probably education. Education should be targeted equally at children, teenagers, and those in the vicinity (parents, school officials, and youth leaders), particularly in situations whereby potential risks for injuries exist. Information should be given on how to avoid injuries and on how to manage them, preferably at the site of the injury. It should be the

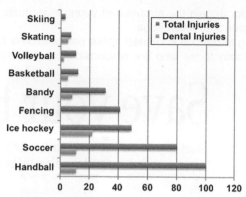

Fig. 2. Dental injuries related to various sports, based on Norwegian insurance records. *Data from* Nysether S. [Traumatic dental injuries among Norwegian athletes]. Nor Tannlaegeforen Tid 1987;97(12):512–4.

aim of every dentist to discuss risk factors that could lead to dental or oral injury during routine dental visits. This education should be aimed at both genders equally. Even though some older epidemiologic data indicated that boys were more prone to sustain oral and dental injury, with increased participation of girls in traditionally male sports (eg, basketball and soccer), as well as in leisure activities (eg, roller-blades and skate-boarding), the gap seems to be narrowing, at least in some geographic areas.[4]

Special strategic measures should be attempted for individuals at high risk, such as those with severe maxillary overjet, as it has been shown that the odds of sustaining dental trauma are significantly and linearly related to the severity of the overjet.[5,6] It has even been suggested that a preventive orthodontic treatment should be initiated for these individuals to be completed before the age of 11 years, that is, in the early to middle mixed dentition stage, in an attempt to reduce their risk of sustaining trauma.[7]

In addition, it is advisable to give special counseling to individuals who present a history of previous oral trauma, as those seem more likely to sustain a new injury compared with those who have not sustained any.[8,9] The risk of sustaining multiple injuries has been reported as being 8.4 times higher when the first trauma episode occurred at 9 years of age, compared with it occurring at age 12.[9] Therefore, young children should receive special attention. Their activities, games, and sports involvement should be carefully assessed, and any risky behavior should be discussed with them, their parents, or those who care for them. A typical example is the recent popularity of basketball hoops that can be lowered from standard height, so that 10- to 12-year-olds can "slam-dunk" or place the ball in the net by jumping up and hanging on the net ring that holds the net after letting go of the ball. Because their arms are short at that age, their maxillary incisors are often at the level of the basket. This scenario has now been reported to result in increasing severities of dental trauma whereby multiple teeth are frequently avulsed.[10]

Information campaigns, whether through television or newspapers, or with distribution of brochures and posters, are also useful strategies for the prevention of traumatic dental injuries. All children should be made aware of correct first aid when an injury occurs. Elements like trying to replant an avulsed tooth immediately or alternatively storing it in milk, and looking for all fragments of a broken tooth before running home for help, should be explained to them in clear, simple language. Posters such as the one sponsored by the International Association of Dental Traumatology

(IADT) and others (**Fig. 3**) gain the attention of young individuals and, if widely displayed, should reinforce their knowledge.

Not only the young should be educated about dental trauma but also those who care for them, especially those who are responsible for their safety during school

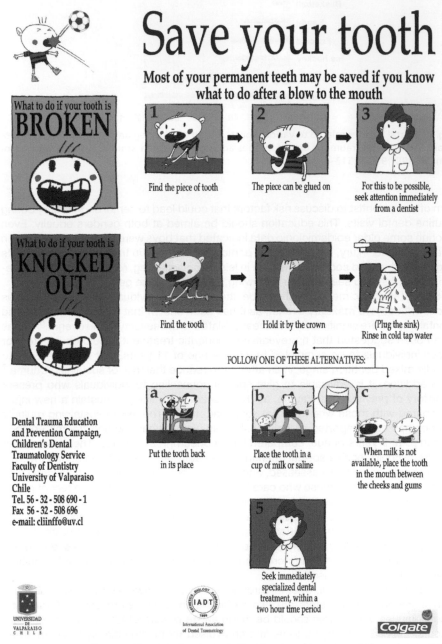

Fig. 3. Poster cosponsored by several national dental organizations and the International Association of Dental Traumatology. (*Courtesy of* The International Association of Dental Traumatology; with permission.)

and organized activities. A simple instruction sheet (**Table 1**) is in most cases sufficient to ensure that injured patients receive proper emergency care at the site of the injury. When educating persons not trained in dentistry it is important to avoid using complicated language. **Table 1** suggests a communication form, which is based on the IADT's guidelines. Its language is clear, and explains in simple terms what to do and what not to do immediately after dental trauma. The form also advises as to the urgency of a necessary dental consultation.

APPLIANCES TO PREVENT DENTAL INJURIES

Traumatic impacts provoke an acute delivery of energy that is released upon soft and hard tissues, resulting in laceration, contusion, or ablation of tissues. Protective devices (eg, mouthguards) to reduce the consequences of such impacts can act by preventing the impact from reaching the oral region or by cushioning, absorbing, or distributing the impact forces. During sports and other activities in which there is a risk of falling or being hit by an object, wearing a faceguard or mouthguard still seems to be the only way to prevent or at least significantly reduce the seriousness of dental injuries. It has been reported that before the mandate of wearing faceguards and mouthguards in United States high school football, facial and oral injuries constituted up to 50% of all reported football injuries.[11,12] Subsequent to the mandate a significant decrease was noted in reported injuries, down to a few percent.[11,13] Another common mechanism of oral injury is traffic accidents. Wearing seatbelts in a car, and using a helmet with a chin arch when riding a motorcycle is mandatory in many countries. Most commonly used bicycling helmets provide good protection against head injuries, as shown in Victoria, Australia when after 1 year of mandatory use of helmets, there was a 48% reduction of reported head injuries in cyclists.[14] Unfortunately these same helmets do not offer any mouth or dental protection.

Faceguards

A faceguard is usually a prefabricated cage of metal or composite that is attached to a helmet or a head strap (**Fig. 4**). Guards made of clear polycarbonate plastic have recently become available, either as prefabricated or custom made. These faceguards seem to provide good protection to the face and teeth, but are not applicable to all activities, and in many cases do not protect the teeth if the individual is hit under the chin.

Few large-scale studies have been conducted on the actual benefits of wearing faceguards in games or practice, but it is clear that the introduction of mandatory helmet and facial protection has been effective in virtually eliminating ocular, facial, and dental injuries in juvenile hockey.[15] However, an unforeseen problem has been reported for the same group of youths: whereas the number of head injuries has been reduced, an increase in catastrophic spinal injuries has been noted. It has been speculated that players get a false sense of security when donning the equipment, leading them to take excessive and unwarranted risks due to the protection they are supposedly afforded.[15] One of the few intervention studies on the effectiveness of faceguards was performed by Danis and colleagues[16] on a group of youth league baseball teams in the United States. Approximately one-half of the teams were supplied with guard helmets (intervention); all others used this protection at their discretion (comparison). The investigators found that the intervention teams reported a reduction in the incidence of oculofacial injuries compared with comparison team respondents ($P = .04$). Half facemasks have been popular in hockey, as it has been speculated that a full face shield may increase the risk of concussions and

Table 1
Suggested review chart for athletic trainees or those responsible for children and teenagers in play

Term	Type of Injury	Immediate Treatment	Dental Referral
Uncomplicated crown fracture	Portion of the tooth broken off No bleeding from the fracture	None	Within 48 hours, especially if the patient has difficulty due to cold sensitivity
Complicated crown fracture	Portion of the tooth broken off and bleeding from the fracture	None; do not place any medication on the bleeding pulp. If needed have the patient bite into a gauge	As soon as logistically possible; could wait until the next morning if the patient tolerates eating and drinking
Root fracture	Tooth might appear in normal position but bleeding from the gum around the tooth The crown of the tooth might be pushed back or loose	None	As soon as possible
Tooth concussion and subluxation	Tooth still in its normal place and firm or slightly loose	None	Within 48 hours, for evaluation only
Luxation	Tooth very loose and/or the crown has moved from its normal position	Only move the tooth back to normal position if it is easy to move it	As soon as possible, especially if it is not possible to reposition the tooth
Avulsion	Tooth completely out of the mouth	Replace the tooth in its hole. If not possible store the tooth in milk or saline	Immediately. It is extremely important for prognosis of the tooth to be treated immediately

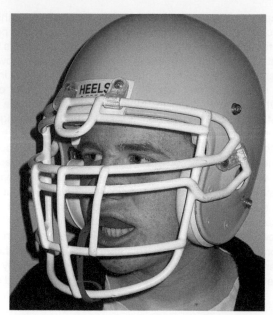

Fig. 4. A typical cagelike face mask as worn by American football players. The mask provides good protection to the face and mouth, but provides minimal protection from a blow under the chin. Note that the athlete is not wearing the mandatory chinstrap.

neck injuries, offsetting the benefits of protection from dental, facial, and ocular injuries. A recent study found that the use of full face shields is associated with a significantly reduced risk of sustaining facial and dental injuries without an increase in the risk of neck injuries, concussions, or other injuries.[17]

With the emergence of many new fiber composites, custom-fabricated faceguards will become easily available and affordable. Studies confirming their benefits must be conducted.

Mouthguards

The use of mouthguards in contact sports has been reported in the past to reduce the occurrence of dental injuries up to 90% or more.[18–21] Because rules regarding the use of headgear and mouthguards in high school football were established in the 1960s, facial and dental injuries sustained on the field have dropped by approximately 48%.[13]

Few studies have specifically investigated, prospectively or in real time, whether athletes who wear mouthguards sustain significantly fewer dental injuries than those who do not.[22–24] The first study to do so involved a sample population of 272 high school rugby players. The athletes received a preseason clinical examination by a team of dentists and completed a questionnaire. Mouthguards were fitted 1 week later and the players were instructed in their use. At the end of the season, a follow-up questionnaire was completed. There was a significant difference in the number of tooth fractures between mouthguard wearers and those without mouthguards. The second study, which evaluated United States male college basketball players (age 18–22 years), collected real-time data. Trainers reported information about their teams on a weekly basis using an interactive Web site. The results of this study are likely to be significant, as it captured 70,936 athlete exposures (an athletic exposure is a one athlete participating in a game or practice, whether it was one play, one quarter, one half, or the entire game). The study found that mouthguard users had significantly lower rates of dental injuries and dentist referrals than nonusers. However, there was no significant difference between mouthguard users and nonusers in the rate of soft tissue injuries. Of note, this study reported significantly more oral or dental injuries than reported by the National Collegiate Athletic Association for the same season.[23] In a more recent study, trainees participating in basic military training at Fort Leonard Wood, Missouri, who were not wearing mouthguards during certain training exercises (eg, unarmed combat, rifle/bayonet training, confidence/obstacle course) were significantly (almost twice) more likely to sustain orofacial injury compared with another group of trainees who were required to wear a mouthguard during all exercises.[24] Not all studies have demonstrated a beneficial effect of mouthguards. In a cross-sectional study, a sample of 321 university rugby players participating on 555 player occasions was examined.[25] The results of that study indicated no statistically significant association between oral, dental, and lip injuries sustained during rugby playing with the use or nonuse of mouthguards. This study, like most mouthguard studies irrespective whether they demonstrated a beneficial effect, is relatively small and therefore likely to have only limited statistical power. Large-scale studies are therefore needed.

Role of mouthguards

It has been suggested that a mouthguard should protect the wearer against injuries in five different ways:[26]

- Preventing tooth injuries by absorbing and deflecting blows to the teeth
- Shielding the lips, tongue, and gingival tissues from laceration
- Preventing opposing teeth from coming into violent contact
- Providing the mandible with resilient support, which absorbs an impact that might fracture the unsupported angle or condyle of the mandible
- Preventing neck and cerebral brain injuries

Various materials and methods have been used in attempts to achieve these basic protective functions of mouthguards; and as many test protocols and devices have been tried to confirm their effectiveness. The main problem with testing mouthguards' eventual protective role is that there is no in vivo model ethically feasible, and in vitro models are at best crude approximations. To further complicate matters, large prospective cohort studies, which could be useful in reaching higher statistical significance, are difficult to conduct and are, to some degree, equally unethical, due to the need for crossover or control groups.

Although no conclusions can be drawn so far from the literature confirming that mouthguards are effective in protecting the wearer, some elements are worth noting:

- In recent studies from a Japanese group an attempt was made to investigate actual objects that could hit mouthguards and teeth during an athletic event, rather than a steel drop-ball that has been frequently used in studies on mouthguards.[27] These studies indicated that transmitted forces were less when a standard single-layer mouthguard was used compared with no mouthguard but, just as important, they demonstrated that the effect was significantly influenced by the object type. The steel ball showed the biggest (62.1%) absorption ability whereas the wooden bat showed the second biggest (38.3%). Other objects, baseball, field hockey ball, and hockey puck, showed from 0.6% to 6.0%

absorbency. These results show that it is important to test the effectiveness of mouthguards on specific types of sports equipment rather than using standard experimental equipment that may provide an unrealistic outcome.

- It has been shown that the physical and mechanical properties vary with their chemical composition, and this itself varies with different brands of the same material (see later in this article). The resilience of PVAc-PE materials seems to vary inversely with the magnitude of the impact energy at which they are tested. Several factors may be responsible for this variation, including the degree of crosslinking between polymer chains, the proportion of plasticizer present, and the volume of filler particles.
- It has been suggested that laminated thermoplastic mouthguards are dimensionally more stable in use.[28]
- It has been suggested that high-energy absorption does not necessarily indicate that the material will give maximum protection, because some of the absorbed energy may be transmitted directly to the underlying dental structures.[29] Research elucidating this matter is needed.

The fifth suggested protective role of a mouthguard is to prevent neck or cerebral brain injuries. Through the years there has been a great deal of discussion in the literature on whether mouthguards contribute toward prevention of cerebral concussion in athletes.[30–32] However, most of the articles have been solely case reports or opinions, unfortunately not based on controlled scientific studies. The two articles usually cited as a foundation of this presumed preventive effect were written by Stenger and colleagues[33] in 1964 and Hickey and colleagues[34] in 1967, both of which are based on limited research and extremely small sample size. With careful scrutiny of scientific evidence in the literature, this claim of protectiveness of the mouthguard on cerebral injuries has been called into serious question.[35] Two large studies using an interactive Web site to collect weekly information on incidence of cerebral brain concussion in athletes have failed to show any benefits.[23,36] In the first study, a comparison was made between those who wore a mouthguard and those who did not in US College men's basketball. Almost 71,000 athletic exposures were reported, but there was no significant difference in the rate of brain concussion between the groups.[23] The second study compared boil-and-bite versus custom-made mouthguards worn by American college football players.[36] More than 500,000 athletic exposures were recorded but again, there was no significant difference between the two groups. These two studies did not assess the mechanism of injury, for example, blow under the chin versus fall to the ground. However and unfortunately, these two studies do not indicate that wearing a mouthguard helps to reduce cerebral brain concussion in any significant way. Manufacturers of stock mouthguards have in recent years started to make unsubstantiated claims regarding their product, and have even gone as far as to market stock mouthguards under brand names like "Brain Pad" and "Brain Pad plus." A study compared the effectiveness of one of these padded dual-jaw mouthguards, the Wipss Brain Pad (Wipss Products Inc., Conshohocken, PA) with other currently used mouthguards in the prevention of concussion injuries in athletes participating in university football and rugby.[37] The study design was a multicenter, cluster-randomized, controlled trial including five Canadian universities for one season. No dental trauma events occurred. The researcher found no significant difference in the concussion rates between players who wore the Wipss Brain Pad mouth guard and those who wore other types of mouthguard. Of note is that no dental injury was reported in the study group during the observation time.[37]

Types of mouthguards
Mouthguards can be divided into 3 basic types based on how they are manufactured and used:

- Stock prefabricated
- Mouth formed
- Custom made

Some of these basic types now have several subgroups, especially the custom-made ones.

- *Stock* mouthguards may be made from rubber or plastic materials. Stock mouthguards are generally available in 2 or 3 sizes; and are supposed to have a universal fit, sometimes aided by flanges in the molar area. Modification is limited to trimming the margins to relieve the frenula. The loose fit means that the wearer must occlude to prevent the guard from being displaced. The main advantage of this type of mouthguard is that they are inexpensive and may be purchased by the public in sports shops. Also, because they do not require any preparation, a replacement is readily available. Most reports agree[38,39] that these types of mouthguard provide the least protection of all available types due to their poor fit, though admittedly there is no conclusive scientific data confirming this opinion. However, it is unquestioned that these mouthguards are uncomfortable for the wearers; they tend to obstruct speech and breathing because the wearer literally must keep them in place by clenching or supporting it with his or her tongue.[40] Therefore they are less likely to be worn and when needed, could be blown out of the mouth before impact with the ground or other obstacles.
- There are two types of *mouth-formed* mouthguards that may be made from a manufactured kit. The first consists of a hard and fairly rigid outer shell that provides a smooth, durable surface and a soft, resilient lining that is adapted to the teeth (**Fig. 5**). The outer shell of vinyl chloride may be lined with a layer of self-curing methyl-methacrylate or silicone rubber. The outer shell is fitted and trimmed, if necessary, around the sulci and frenal attachments. The shell is filled with the soft lining and seated in the mouth. Care must be taken to ensure that it is centrally placed. The lining is allowed to polymerize for 3 to 5 minutes. Excess material is trimmed with a sharp knife, and the margins smoothed with dental stones. This type of mouthguard tends to be bulky, and the margins of the outer shell may be sharp unless protected by an adequate thickness of the lining material. The most commonly used type of mouth-formed protector is constructed from a preformed thermoplastic shell of PVAc-PE copolymer or PVC[38] that is softened in warm water and then molded in the mouth by the user (see **Fig. 5**). These mouthguards have several distinct advantages over the stock mouthguard. If carefully adapted, they give a closer fit and are more easily retained than stock protectors. Care must be taken during the molding process so that the mouthguard fits accurately. The temperature necessary to allow adequate adaptation to the teeth is fairly high, so additional care must be taken to avoid burning the gingiva. Similar to the stock mouthguard, this type of mouthguard is relatively inexpensive, readily available to the general public, and can be formed into a decent appliance with some care.
- *Custom* mouthguards are individually made in a laboratory, on plaster of Paris models poured from impressions of the player's mouth. Many studies have shown that these mouthguards are more acceptable and comfortable to athletes than the other types[41,42] There is no evidence, however, that custom-made protectors are

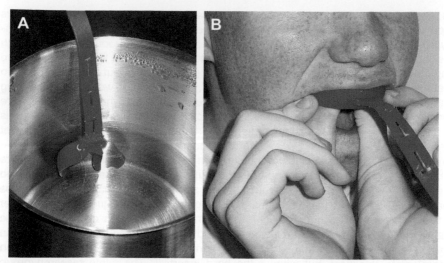

Fig. 5. Boil-and-bite being formed in the mouth. (*A*) The stock mouthguard is heated in boiling water and then inserted in the mouth. (*B*) The index fingers are used to adapt the mouthguard as well as possible to the facial sides of the molars, while the thumbs press on the palatal side.

more effective in preventing injuries. Historically, three groups of materials have been used to fabricate custom-made mouth protectors: molded velum rubber,[41] latex rubber,[43] and resilient acrylic resins. By far the most common material being used currently for custom-made mouthguards is ethylene vinyl acetate (EVA) copolymers. Polyvinylchloride and soft acrylic resins such as polyurethane were also used previously, but the superiority of the EVA copolymers has practically eliminated the others. Its popularity is mainly due to its elastomeric softness and flexibility, and it can be relatively easily processed. Also, the material has good clarity and gloss, barrier properties, low-temperature toughness, stress-crack resistance, and little or no odor.[38,44] Many prefabricated plates of EVA are now commercially available; but it is important to know that the percentage of vinyl acetate (often marked %) can vary between manufacturers, therefore the plates can show different properties. When higher proportions of vinyl acetate are copolymerized (higher % marking), the EVA plate is more flexible, stretchable, softer, and tougher.[44] This higher percentage also lowers the softening temperature, allowing manipulation of the material within a comfortable temperature. The most common EVA copolymers used for fabrication of mouthguards contain 28% vinyl acetate. It should be remembered, though, that the actual performance of a mouthguard relies not only on its intrinsic material properties but also on its design and thickness, and on the type of traumatic impact on the mouth.[44]

The EVA mouthguard material can be bought in varying colors, thickness, and hardness. There has been discussion on whether there should be a different stiffness or hardness for different sports. Thus, whereas the low-stiffness guards absorb shock during hard-object collisions (eg, baseballs), they may not protect the tooth bone during soft-object collisions (eg, boxing gloves).[45] To date, clinical studies to substantiate such recommendations are lacking.

In 1985 Chaconas and colleagues[28] described a laminated thermoplastic mouthguard that showed significantly less dimensional change than other materials tested (ie, poly(vinyl acetate-ethylene) copolymer clear thermoplastic, polyurethane). This type was the first of several different subcategories within custom-made mouthguards. A few years ago, layered EVA stock plates were introduced (**Fig. 6**), with the intention of further strengthening the mouthguard without losing its protective capacity. When a stock plate of EVA is fabricated, it is drawn out in one direction so that the polymer chains are more or less parallel, like the grain in wood. This stretching can theoretically make a difference to the plate's properties whether the grains are running faciopalatally or mesiodistally on the crown of the tooth. To eliminate this and increase the stiffness without adding bulk, manufacturers have started to market two- or three-layered stock EVA, whereby the layers have been added perpendicular to each other. Some manufacturers have even added a low-percentage EVA plate between layers, which is designed to further stiffen the mouthguard palatally behind the anterior incisors. There is not much, if any, scientific proof that this can increase the protectiveness of the mouthguard and again raises the question of whether a too stiff mouthguard could cause other damage to the teeth or alveolus. Some alarming findings were reported in a recent study.[46] A hard insert resulted in reduced energy absorption when compared with a control sheet of the same material and approximate thickness but without the hard inserts.[46] The same research group has, however, shown improved impact characteristics of the EVA mouthguard material with regulated air inclusions.[47] However, as yet there are no clinical data available to support this finding, and durability of air-included mouthguards is unknown.

Another version of this layered concept is the fusion of two plates of different stiffness. However, these plates only seem to improve the mouthguard when the softer material is next to the teeth. A study by Kim and Mathieu,[29] using a finite element model, showed that a soft outer layer covering a hard core had no significant difference from a monolayer in stress distribution and impact force. However, a soft core was found to have a significant effect on stress distribution. This effect could be increased by controlling ratios of modulus and volume fractions of the core and outer layer.

The main question regarding these various types of mouthguards is whether there is any actual protective difference between them. Few studies have investigated the efficacy of the different types in preventing dental injuries with large enough samples to have significant power. In one study on 98 professional rugby players, custom-made mouthguards did not significantly reduce the amount of dental injuries sustained compared with mouth-formed mouthguards.[48] At a follow-up clinical examination, there was no damage to teeth when either custom-made or boil-and-bite mouthguards were worn. Stokes and colleagues[41] compared mouth-formed and custom-made mouthguards. This study showed that although there were no dental injuries in either group, the users preferred laboratory-formed mouthguards for reasons of comfort. In a large study on college football players, trainers reported data every

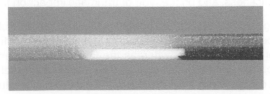

Fig. 6. Prefabricated double-layered mouthguard stock plate. Both layers contain the same percentage of vinyl acetate, but the top layer is clear and the bottom layer is composed of three different colors, all fused into one mass, for aesthetic reasons.

week for the entire season, through an interactive Web site, on the number of players, mouthguard use, and dental and oral injuries. There was no apparent difference reported between boil-and-bite or custom-made mouthguards.[49] The sample consisted of 87 (76%) of a possible 114 Division I teams, with a total of 506,297 athletic exposures recorded. Most of the teams used a mixture of custom and boil-and-bite mouthguards, so there was a possibility that the benefits of one particular mouthguard might not be clearly defined. Therefore, the data were further analyzed whereby a subselection of 14 teams were selected, 7 of which used exclusively custom-made mouthguards and the other 7, exclusively boil-and-bite. The results were the same, as no statistically significant benefit of one type of mouthguard was found over the other.[49] It is important to stress that in this study there was no attempt to inspect the quality of the mouthguard used or the comfort of one type over the other. One more recent study does, however, indicate that there might be some difference.[50] In that study Australian Rules football community teams were randomly allocated to use either a custom-made mouthguard or stock mouthguard during games. The results showed that there was a significant protective effect of custom-made mouthguards, relative to using stock mouthguards. However, the study reported on head and oral injures combined, not solely on dental injuries. Also, it lacked a control group.[50]

Wear and tear affects all mouthguards; and it has been suggested that they should be replaced regularly not only due to lack of fit but also because of reduction in protective properties. It has been shown recently in a simulated aging study on different types of custom-made mouthguards that aging induced various dimensional changes. Most of the dimensional changes for all types of mouthguards occurred at the central incisor region. However, pressure-laminated mouthguard specimens showed the lowest range of changes at the central incisor region, suggesting potentially improved fit, comfort, and protection.[51]

Fabrication of mouthguards

Organizations such as the Federation Dentaire International (FDI)[52] have created and published recommended criteria on the construction of an effective mouthguard. Most of these recommendations state the same things:

1. The mouthguard should be made of a resilient material, which can be easily washed and cleaned, and readily disinfected.
2. It should have adequate retention to remain in position during sporting activity, and allow for a normal occlusal relationship to give maximum protection.
3. It should absorb and disperse the energy of a shock by:
   • Covering the maxillary dental arch
   • Excluding interference
   • Reproducing the occlusal relationship
   • Allowing mouth breathing
   • Protecting the soft tissues

Furthermore, the FDI also recommends that mouthguards be made by dentists from an impression of the athlete's teeth.

Fabrication of a mouth-formed mouthguard Regardless of type, the key for functionality is selection of a stock that fits the arch. If too small, it is likely that the molars will not be properly covered, thereby reducing retention and fit (**Fig. 7**). Once the proper size is found and fitted, the mouthguard should be made strictly following the manufacturer's guidelines or recommendations.

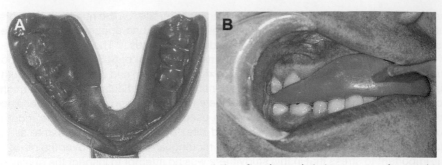

Fig. 7. (*A*) Selection of a stock mouthguard that fits the arch is important when making a boil-and-bite mouthguard. (*B*) If the stock is too small, the molar area will be insufficiently covered, thus reducing retention and fit.

Fabrication of a custom-made mouthguard The best way to construct a custom mouthguard is to take alginate impressions of both arches together with a wax bite taken with the patient's mandible in a physiologic rest position. However, when time and cost is a major issue, an impression of the maxilla can be considered sufficient. It is important to get a good impression of the alveolus over all teeth, even to the point that the vestibule is overextended (**Fig. 8**). This impression will allow good adaptation of the mouthguard material to the soft tissue area, and will in turn ensure better retention and comfort. In a crossover study of different mouthguard extensions, McClelland and colleagues[53] found that comfort of wear was likely to be increased if the mouthguard was extended labially to within 2 mm of the vestibular fold, adjusted to allow even occlusal contact, rounded at the buccal peripheries, and tapered at the palatal edges. To further ensure good adaptation of the mouthguard material to the cast, the cast should be carefully trimmed so the vestibule is almost removed (**Fig. 9**). It has also been shown that residual moisture in the working cast is the most critical factor in determining the fit of the mouthguard made by vacuum-forming machines. The best fit was achieved when the working cast was thoroughly dried and its surface temperature was elevated.[54]

There are two basic methods of fabricating a custom-made mouthguard. The first uses the more traditional vacuum suction machine (**Fig. 10**) that basically draws the EVA stock plate over the plaster cast. It is possible to use either the single-layer or

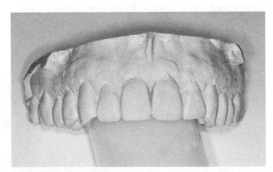

Fig. 8. The impression should include not only the teeth but also the alveolar tissues up to the vestibule, especially in the anterior region (as seen reflected in this cast). This shape will allow proper adaptation of the mouthguard to the soft tissue area, thus ensuring better retention.

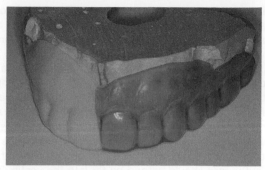

Fig. 9. The cast should be trimmed so that the vestibule is almost removed, ensuring a good adaptation of the mouthguard material to the cast when it is sucked over the cast.

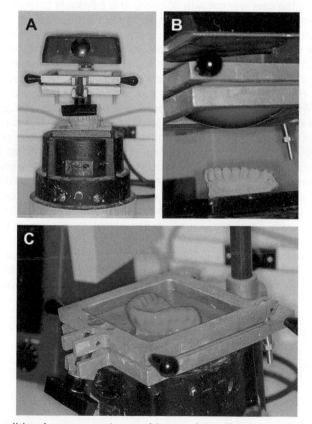

Fig. 10. (*A*) A traditional vacuum suction machine used to make custom-made mouthguards. At the top is the heating element. The stock plate is sandwiched in a jig directly underneath the heating element. The cast is placed and centered on a perforated plate. (*B*) When the stock plate heats up it will start to drop. Care must be taken not to overheat it because this will result in a mouthguard that is too thin. Most commonly used EVA materials should drop about 2 to 2.5 cm (0.75 to 1 inch). (*C*) Before it is removed from the cast, the plate needs to cool down completely.

prefabricated multilayered EVA in these machines; but it is difficult to create a multila-minated mouthguard from separate plates using this technique, as adaptation of layers will always be poor. There is a high risk of the mouthguard coming apart during use and its benefit is thus lost.

There are several critical steps that must be followed when this type of mouthguard is made. The first step is to drill a hole in the palatal area of the cast to improve the suction and thereby adaptation (**Fig. 11**), to ensure good suction in the palatal region. The second step is to allow the heated EVA plate to adapt well to the cast and cool in place. If the formed mouthguard is removed while still warm there is great risk of deformation, which will result in poor adaptation to the teeth and surrounding tissue and thereby poor retention. The third step is proper trimming of the mouthguard after it has cooled completely. The mouthguard should extend as far into the vestibule as tolerated by the patient, with appropriate clearance of the buccal and labial frenula. It should extend as far back on the palate as reasonable to increase anterior strength and retention (**Fig. 12**).[53] The mouthguard should cover at least up to the second molar distally (**Fig. 13**).[55] The mouthguard can be trimmed with a specially heated knife on the cast or removed from the cast and cut with scissors. It is advisable to replace the mouth-guard on the cast after trimming is complete, and to flame the edges with a torch. Alter-natively, the edges can be smoothed with a small rag-wheel in a hand trimmer. To further improve the athlete's comfort, it is possible to gently heat the occlusal surface and then have the athlete bite together with the guard in place; this can also be done on an articulator, if casts of both arches and bite registration have been made.

The second method of fabrication of a custom-made mouthguard uses positive pressure machines, such as Drufomat, Erkopress-2004, or Biostar. In these machines, the stock plate is pressed, after being heated, onto the cast with pressure from above the plate rather than being drawn down onto the cast with negative pressure from below. This action will ensure close adaptation of the material to the cast, and it is rela-tively easy to add multiple layers, as the positive pressure will always ensure that the new layer adapts to the existing one. Thus, the stiffness of the mouthguard can quickly build up with the multiple layers, but without losing adaptation to the teeth. However, there must be some resilience in the mouthguard, so care must be taken not to make the appliance too stiff. This technique offers the advantage of allowing the sandwich-ing of names, numbers, or logos between layers.

The mouthguard should then be inspected for quality and thickness. Some effort has been made to find the ideal thickness to ensure comfort as well as to yield optimal protection. The consensus seems to be that the thicker the mouthguard, the more

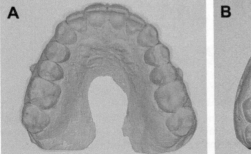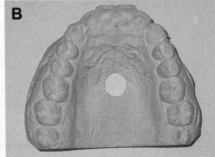

Fig. 11. (*A, B*) Drilling a hole or trimming the palatal area of the cast is necessary to improve the suction and thereby adaptation. Trimming is feasible only for individuals with a high palatal vault, because otherwise lies the danger of removing too much of the alveolar process.

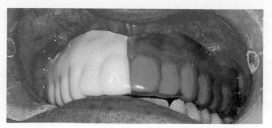

Fig.12. The mouthguard should extend as far up in the vestibule as tolerated by the patient, but with appropriate clearance of the buccal and labial frenulum.

protection it yields. However, if thickness exceeds 4 mm, it seems performance is improved only marginally and the mouthguard becomes less comfortable for the wearer.[42,56]

Common pitfalls in fabricating custom-made mouthguards include the following.
1. Extension above the teeth:
   The more the gums are covered above the teeth, the greater the retention.
     Mouthguard's strength increases as well.
   Overextension is uncomfortable and could lead to injury in the vestibule.
   The mouthguard should be trimmed so that the frenulum is free.
2. Extension over the molar area:
   The mouthguard should cover at least one molar tooth on each side.
   Some extension over the gums in the molar region is recommended for retention.
3. Extension in the palatal area:
   The mouthguard needs to cover some of the tissue above and behind the anterior
     teeth.
   This fit will increase retention and strength of the mouthguard.
4. Rough edges:
   Rough edges are uncomfortable and cause additional injuries.
   They should be smoothed with a flame, sandpaper, or rag-wheel.
5. Too thin or too thick:

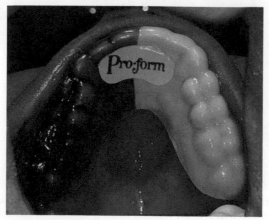

Fig. 13. The mouthguard should extend as far back as reasonable on the palate, to increase anterior strength and retention; distally, it should ideally cover up to the second molar at least.

mouthguard that isoo thin will not be strong enough to provide protection. mouthguard that istoo thick will be uncomfortable to wear.

Use of mouthguards: indications

Mouthguards can strategically be used as preventive appliances for traumatic dental injuries during practice of various sports activities, such as American football, baseball, basketball, boxing, field and ice hockey, and rugby, even though their protective role remains questionable. The mouthguard should be properly connected to the facemask or helmet (**Fig. 14**).

Alternatively, mouthguards seem to offer protection of the dental tissues during general anesthesia. Indeed, oral endoscopy and orotracheal intubation may result in fracture or displacement of teeth.[57–59] Damage may be inflicted by using the incisal edges of the anterior teeth as a fulcrum when inserting a laryngoscope, retractors, or endoscopes. The fracture of prosthetic crowns has also been reported, and injuries to the teeth are one of the most frequent complications during the delivery of general anesthesia.[60] However, it is not clear how frequent this kind of trauma is, for it is likely that in many cases the damage is not discovered until months if not years later, because the tooth or teeth only sustained mild luxation during the trauma rather than crown fracture or frank avulsion. Custom-made mouthguards have not been considered cost effective, which might be in part because anesthesiologists fear that the mouthguard could get in the way during intubation. However, a recent study showed that when comparing the intubation time of 80 patients, half of whom had a mouthguard and the other half did not, there was on average only a 7 seconds difference between the two groups.[61] If one considers the possible cost of legal action due to dental trauma, even as infrequent as it may be, the case for any type of dental protection during intubation becomes even stronger. In addition, in situations in which there is a great risk of

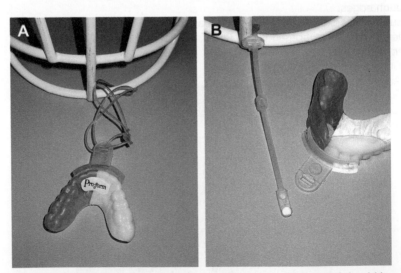

Fig. 14. The connection between a facemask or helmet and a mouthguard should have self-releasing mechanisms so that if those happen to be propelled off the athlete following an impact, a forceful pull on the mouthguard (which can damage the teeth or the dental arch) is prevented. (*A*) The mouthguard should never be tied to the facemask or other appliances that could come loose. (*B*) A special releasing attachment should be used instead.

complications due to restorations, limited mouth opening, and so forth, the use of a protective dental appliance constitutes an advisable and strategic preventive approach.[62,63]

REFERENCES

1. Peterson EE, Andersson L, Sörensen S. Traumatic oral vs non-oral injuries. An epidemilogical study during one year in a Swedish county. Swed Dent J 1997; 21:55–68.
2. Skaare AB, Jacobsen I. Etiological factors related to dental injuries in Norwegians aged 7–18 years. Dent Traumatol 2003;19:304–8.
3. Andreasen FM. "The price of a blue tooth—the cost of dental trauma" presented at the World Congress on Sports Dentistry and Dental Traumatology. Boston, USA. June 20–24, 2001.
4. Gutmann JK, Gutmann MS. Cause, incidence, and prevention of trauma to teeth. Dent Clin North Am 1995;39:1–13.
5. Eichenbaum I. A correlation of traumatised anterior teeth to occlusion. ASDC J Dent Child 1963;30:229–36.
6. Shulman JD, Peterson J. The association between incisor trauma and occlusal characteristics in individuals 8-50 years of age. Dent Traumatol 2004;20:67–74.
7. Bauss A, Röhling J, Schwetka-Polly R. Prevalence of traumatic injuries to the permanent incisors in candidates for orthodontic treatment. Dent Traumatol 2004;20:61–6.
8. Glendor UB. On dental trauma in children and adolescents. Incidence, risk, treatment, time and costs. Swed Dent J Suppl 2000;140:1–52.
9. Glendor UB, Koucheki B, Halling A. Risk evaluation and type of treatment of multiple dental trauma episodes to permanent teeth. Endod Dent Traumatol 2000;165:205–10.
10. Kumamoto DP, Winter J, Novickas D, et al. Tooth avulsions resulting from basketball net entanglement. J Am Dent Assoc 1997;128:1273–5.
11. Heintz WD. Mouth protectors: a progress report. Bureau of Dental Health Education. J Am Dent Assoc 1968;77:632–6.
12. Bureau of Dental Health Education. Mouth protectors: 11 years later. J Am Dent Assoc 1973;86:1365.
13. Gabon MA, Wright JT. Mouth protectors and oral trauma: a study of adolescent football players. J Am Dent Assoc 1986;112:663–5.
14. Vulcan AP, Cameron MH, Watson WL. Mandatory bicycle helmet use, experience in Victoria, Australia. World J Surg 1992;16:389–97.
15. Murray TM, Livingston A. Hockey helmets, face masks, and injurious behavior. Pediatrics 1995;95:419–21.
16. Danis RP, Hu K, Bell M. Acceptability of baseball face guards and reduction of oculofacial injury in receptive youth league players. Inj Prev 2000;6:232–4.
17. Benson BW, Mohtadi NG, Rose MS, et al. Head and neck injuries among ice hockey players wearing full face shields vs half face shields. J Am Med Assoc 1999;282:2328–32.
18. Davies RM, Bradley D, Hale RW, et al. The prevalence of dental injuries in rugby players and their attitude to mouthguards. Br J Sports Med 1977;11:72–4.
19. Hugston JC. Prevention of dental injuries in sports. Am J Sports Med 1980;8: 61–2.
20. de Wet FA. The prevention of orofacial sports injuries in the adolescent. Int Dent J 1981;31:313–9.

21. Chapman PJ, Nasser BP. Prevalence of orofacial injuries and use of mouthguards in high school rugby union. Aust Dent J 1996;41:252–5.
22. Morton JG, Burton JF. An evaluation of the effectiveness of mouthguards in high-school rugby players. N Z Dent J 1979;75:151–3.
23. LaBella CR, Smith BW, Sigurdsson A. Effect of mouthguards on dental injuries and concussions in college basketball. Med Sci Sports Exerc 2002;34:41–4.
24. Bourdin M, Brunet-Patru I, Hager PE, et al. Influence of maxillary mouthguards on physiological parameters. Med Sci Sports Exerc 2006;38(8):1500–4.
25. Blignaut JB, Carstens IL, Lombard CJ. Injuries sustained in rugby by wearers and non-wearers of mouthguards. Br J Sports Med 1987;21:5–7.
26. Stevens OO. In: Andreasen JO, editor. Traumatic injuries to the teeth. Copenhagen: Munskgaard; 1981. p. 439–50.
27. Takeda T, Ishigami K, Shintaro K, et al. The influence of impact object characteristics on impact force and force absorption by mouthguard material. Dent Traumatol 2004;20:12–20.
28. Chaconas SJ, Caputo AA, Bakke NK. A comparison of athletic mouthguard materials. Am J Sports Med 1985;13:193–7.
29. Kim HS, Mathieu K. Application of laminates to mouthguards: finite element analysis. J Mater Sci Mater Med 1998;9:457–62.
30. Chapman PJ. The bimaxillary mouthguard: a preliminary report of use in contact sports. Aust Dent J 1986;31:200–6.
31. Chapman PJ. Mouthguard protection in sports. Aust Dent J 1996;41:212.
32. Biasca NS, Wirth S, Tegner Y. The avoidability of head and neck injuries in ice hockey: an historical review. Br J Sports Med 2002;36:410–27.
33. Stenger JM, Lawson E, Wright JM, et al. Mouthguards: protection against shock to head, neck and teeth. J Am Dent Assoc 1964;69:273–81.
34. Hickey JC, Morris AL, Carlson LD, et al. The relation of mouth protectors to cranial pressure and deformation. J Am Dent Assoc 1967;74:735–40.
35. McCrory P. Do mouthguards prevent concussion? Br J Sports Med 2001;35:81–2.
36. Wisniewski JF, Guskiewicz K, Trope M, et al. Incidence of cerebral concussions associated with type of mouthguard used in college football. Dent Traumatol 2004;20:143–9.
37. Barbic D, Pater J, Brison RJ. Comparison of mouth guard designs and concussion prevention in contact sports: a multicenter randomized controlled trial. Clin J Sport Med 2005;15(5):294–8.
38. Going RE, Loehman RE, Chan MS. Mouthguard materials: their physical and mechanical properties. J Am Dent Assoc 1974;89:132–8.
39. ChalmersMouthguards DJ. Protection for the mouth in rugby union. Sports Med 1998;25:339–49.
40. Walker J, Jakobsen J, Brown S. Attitudes concerning mouthguard use in 7- to 8-year-old children. ASDC J Dent Child 2002;69:207–11, 126.
41. Stokes AN, Croft GC, Gee D. Comparison of laboratory and intraorally formed mouth protectors. Endod Dent Traumatol 1987;3:255–8.
42. Chapman PJ. Mouthguard protection in sports injury. Aust Dent J 1995;40:136.
43. Nicholas NK. Mouth protection in contact sports. N Z Dent J 1969;65:14–24.
44. Park JB, Shaull KL, Overton B, et al. Improving mouth guards. J Prosthet Dent 1994;72:373–80.
45. Cummings NK, Spears IR. The effect of mouthguard design on stresses in the tooth-bone complex. Med Sci Sports Exerc 2002;34:942–7.

46. Westerman BP, Stringfellow PM, Eccleston JA. The effect on energy absorption of hard inserts in laminated EVA mouthguards. Aust Dent J 2000;45:21–3.

47. Westerman BP, Stringfellow PM, Eccleston JA. Beneficial effects of air inclusions on the performance of ethylene vinyl acetate EVA mouthguard material. Br J Sports Med 2002;36:51–3.

48. Upson N. Mouthguards, an evaluation of two types for rugby players. Br J Sports Med 1985;19:89–92.

49. Wisniewski JF, Sigurdsson A, Trope M, et al. Cerebral concussions and dental injuries: incidence associated with types of mouthguard worn. J Endod 2003; 29(4):308 [abstract PR 37].

50. Finch C, Braham R, McIntosh A, et al. Should football players wear custom fitted mouthguards? Results from a group randomised controlled trial. Inj Prev 2005; 11(4):242–6.

51. Waked EJ, Lee TK, Caputo AA. Effects of aging on the dimensional stability of custom-made mouthguards. Quintessence Int 2002;33:700–5.

52. Federation Dentaire International, F.D.I. Commission on dental products. Proceedings of the Federation Dentaire Internationale. Working Party No. 7. 1990.

53. McClelland C, Kinirons M, Geary L. A preliminary study of patient comfort associated with customized mouthguards. Br J Sports Med 1999;33:186–9.

54. Yonehata Y, Maeda Y, Machi H, et al. The influence of working cast residual moisture and temperature on the fit of vacuum-forming athletic mouth guards. J Prosthet Dent 2003;89:23–7.

55. Yamanaka T, Ueno T, Oki M, et al. Study on the effects of shortening the distal end of a mouthguard using modal analysis. J Med Dent Sci 2002;49:129–33.

56. Westerman BP, Stringfellow PM, Eccleston JA. EVA mouthguards: how thick should they be? Dent Traumatol 2002;18:24–7.

57. Bamforth BJ. Complications during endotracheal anaesthesia. Anesth Analg 1963;42:727–32.

58. Wright RB, Manfield FFV. Damage to the teeth during the administration of general anaesthesia. Anesth Analg 1974;53:405–8.

59. McCarthy G, Carlson O. A dental splint for use during per oral endoscopy. Acta Otolaryngol 1977;84:450–2.

60. Lockhart PB, Feldbau EV, Babel RA. Dental complications during and after tracheal intubation. J Am Dent Assoc 1986;112:480–3.

61. Brosnan C, Radford P. The effect of a toothguard on the difficulty of intubation. Anaesthesia 1997;52:1011–4.

62. Chadwick RG, Lindsay M. Dental injuries during general anaesthesia. Br Dent J 1996;180:255–8.

63. Skeie A, Schwartz O. Traumatic injuries of the teeth in connection with general anaesthesia and the effect of use of mouthguards. Endod Dent Traumatol 1999;15:33–6.

Trauma Kits for the Dental Office

David E. Jaramillo, DDS*, Leif K. Bakland, DDS

KEYWORDS

• Trauma kit • Dental trauma • Trauma classification

Traumatic dental injuries tend to be unexpected and injured patients typically arrive in the dental office on an emergency basis. They have to be fitted in, often in a busy schedule, and not much time is available to examine, plan procedures, discuss options, and provide treatment. Yet, they need attention, and in some cases, the length of time between accident and treatment is critical for a successful outcome. Therefore, it makes sense that a dental office to which patients with dental injuries may come, would be prepared to provide efficient and correct emergency treatment.

To be well prepared for traumatic dental injuries, it helps to recognize that such injuries vary in terms of urgency for treatment. Andreasen and colleagues[1] have recommended treatment priorities based on the effect of time between accident and treatment. The time frames indicated are for the purpose of predicting best outcomes. Teeth can be treated after the ideal time frame and still experience successful outcomes.

Treatment priorities
1. Acute. Should be treated within a few hours. Injuries include: avulsions, extrusions, lateral luxations, and root fractures.
2. Subacute. Should be treated within 24 hours. Injuries include: intrusions, subluxations, crown fractures with pulp exposure.
3. Delayed. Can be delayed more than 24 hours. Injury: crown fractures without pulp exposure.

An example of triaging an injury based on this categorization would be the case of a complicated crown fracture with pulp exposure. If a patient with such an injury arrives on an emergency basis, a quick temporary covering of the pulp wound with, for example, glass ionomer can protect the exposed pulp and the patient can be treated later that day or the next day.

As with all successful dental procedures, knowledge and preparation are the basis for a successful result. To that end, this article will first classify traumatic dental injuries

Department of Endodontics, School of Dentistry, Loma Linda University, Loma Linda, CA 92354, USA
* Corresponding author.
E-mail address: djaramillo@llu.edu (D.E. Jaramillo).

Dent Clin N Am 53 (2009) 751–760
doi:10.1016/j.cden.2009.06.005
0011-8532/09/$ – see front matter © 2009 Elsevier Inc. All rights reserved.

and assign them to their proper urgency category, and then describe treatment kits that can be prepared for various injuries along with identifying proper treatment in each case. One must keep in mind, though, that combination of injuries may occur; primary attention should be given to the more serious one.

CLASSIFICATION AND TREATMENT PRIORITIES

The emphasis in this article will be dental traumatic injuries involving teeth and the periodontal ligament. Soft tissue injuries (ie, lacerations, contusions, and abrasions) are usually managed in emergency rooms and will not be included here.[1]

Enamel Fractures

Enamel fractures only involve enamel and no urgency exists. Treatment can be performed at any time.

Uncomplicated Crown Fracture

Uncomplicated crown fractures involve enamel and dentin but not the pulp (**Fig. 1**). There is low treatment priority (delayed); outcome is not affected if treatment is delayed more than 24 hours. The tooth should, however, be kept clean to prevent bacterial growth on the exposed dentin surface.

Complicated Crown Fracture

Complicated crown fractures involve enamel, dentin, and pulp (**Fig. 2**). Priority is subacute, which means that treatment should be done as soon as possible, preferably within 24 hours. The pulp, however, can survive for many hours as long as it is healthy. This type of injury can be treated with a pulp cap or shallow pulpotomy. If the tooth is a fully formed tooth in an adult and root canal treatment is chosen, it can be done at a time convenient for the patient and the dentist.

Crown-root Fracture

Crown-root fractures involve enamel, dentin, and cementum, and possibly the pulp (**Fig. 3**). Treatment priority is similar to crown fractures, depending on whether or not the pulp is involved.

Root Fracture

Root fractures involve cementum, dentin, and pulp (**Fig. 4**). They are usually horizontal or diagonal. Treatment priority is acute, particularly if the coronal segment has been

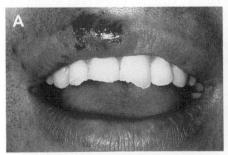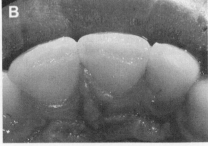

Fig. 1. (*A*) Crown fracture involving enamel and dentin is referred to as an uncomplicated fracture. (*B*) The pulp is not exposed, but bacterial toxins can reach the pulp through exposed dentinal tubules. (*Courtesy of* L. K. Bakland, DDS, Loma Linda, CA.)

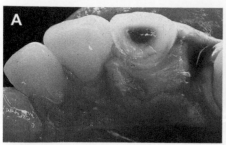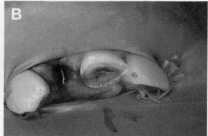

Fig. 2. (*A*) Crown fracture exposing the pulp is referred to as a complicated crown fracture. (*B*) Protecting the pulp will allow healing and continued root formation, which is important in young patients and such procedures should be done under a dental dam. (*Courtesy of* L. K. Bakland, DDS, Loma Linda, CA.)

displaced. Treatment consists of repositioning to coronal segment and stabilizing the tooth for 4 to 6 weeks. Variations in treatment may be dictated by the fracture position; fractures close to the crest of the alveolar bone may benefit from extended splinting periods.

Luxation Injuries

Luxation injuries involve the teeth and the periodontal ligament (PDL), and may also involve the supporting alveolar bone (**Fig. 5**). The injuries can be identified into five categories: concussion, subluxation, extrusive luxation, lateral luxation, and intrusive luxation.

Concussion

Concussion involves the tooth and the PDL. The tooth is painful to percussion, but has not been displaced and healing is usually uneventful, particularly in young patients. No treatment is indicated other than symptomatic attention, such as avoiding biting hard on the tooth until it is comfortable. Monitoring the tooth for possible pulpal deterioration is indicated, particularly in mature, fully developed teeth.

Subluxation

Subluxation involves the tooth, the PDL, and also some minor damage to the supporting alveolar bone. Treatment priority is subacute. The tooth is painful to percussion

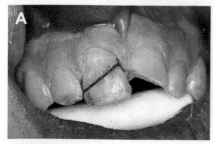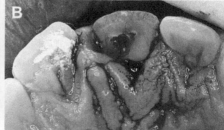

Fig. 3. (*A*) Fracture involving the crown and the root. Often the coronal fragment is still in place because it is attached to periodontal ligament in the root portion. (*B*) Usually in maxillary anterior teeth involved with root fractures, the radicular part of the fracture extends down the root on the apical side of the tooth. The pulp is exposed in this tooth. (*Courtesy of* L. K. Bakland, DDS, Loma Linda, CA.)

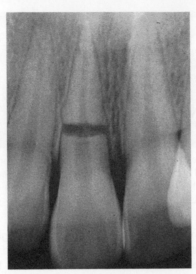

Fig. 4. Horizontal root fracture of a maxillary central incisor. If the coronal segment can be repositioned in good approximation to the apical root segment, healing is quite predictable. (*Courtesy of* L. K. Bakland, DDS, Loma Linda, CA.)

and has increased mobility compared with adjacent uninjured teeth. No treatment is usually needed, but stabilization for a short period of time (ie, 2–4 weeks) will provide patient comfort. Subluxated teeth must be monitored for pulpal deterioration, particularly in mature, fully developed teeth.

Extrusive luxation
Extrusive luxation involves the tooth, the PDL, and possibly the supporting alveolar bone. The tooth will be mobile compared with uninjured adjacent teeth and will probably be sensitive to percussion; it will be partially extruded from the alveolar socket. Treatment consists of repositioning the tooth into its original location and stabilizing the tooth for 4 weeks. Treatment priority is acute. In immature, developing teeth with apical openings greater than 1 mm in diameter, pulpal revascularization is possible, but not

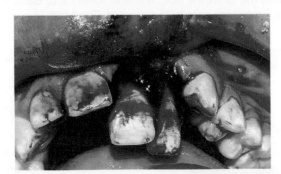

Fig. 5. Luxation injuries range from concussion to intrusive luxation. Frequently, many teeth are involved, each with a different injury. In this patient, the maxillary left central and lateral incisors are laterally luxated (pushed palatally) and quite possibly the adjacent teeth have at least undergone concussion injury and possibly subluxation, making it important to examine adjacent teeth and the obviously injured ones. (*Courtesy of* S. Curiel, DDS Leon, Mexico.)

predictable. In mature fully developed teeth, pulpal revascularization is not expected and root canal therapy is recommended. Endodontic treatment can be initiated 10 to 14 days after the initial emergency treatment of repositioning and splinting.

Lateral luxation
Lateral luxation involves the tooth, the PDL, and the supporting alveolar bone. The tooth has been displaced and often the apical part of the root has been forced into the adjacent bone making the tooth appear ankylosed, without mobility. It is usually not overly painful to percussion. Treatment priority is acute. Treatment consists of re-positioning the tooth into its original position, stabilizing it for 4 weeks, during which time root canal treatment is recommended and can be initiated 10 to 14 days after emergency treatment if the tooth is fully developed. Young, immature teeth have the potential for pulpal revascularization, but it is not predictable.

Intrusive luxation
Intrusive luxation involves the tooth, the PDL, and the supporting alveolar bone. The tooth is completely firm because it has been displaced vertically into the alveolar bone. It appears ankylosed and is usually not painful to percussion. Treatment priority is subacute, but it depends on the patient's age. Children under the age of 15 have the potential for intruded teeth to spontaneously re-erupt. When that happens, the outcome of the traumatic injury leads to the best possible result. In patients over the age of 15, the intruded teeth should be repositioned either orthodontically or surgi-cally, and root canal therapy is recommended. The endodontic treatment can be initi-ated within 10 to 14 days after repositioning the tooth surgically, or as soon as accessible if repositioned orthodontically. After repositioning, regardless of technique, the tooth needs to be stabilized for 4 weeks.[1]

Avulsion

In avulsion, the tooth has been completely ex-articulated from its socket (**Fig. 6**). Treat-ment priority is acute and consists of replanting the tooth in a most timely manner. Ideally, avulsed teeth should be replanted at the site of injury; the outcome is directly related to the time the tooth is away from its normal environment. If the patient, or the person helping the patient, is unable to replant the tooth on site, it can be transported with the patient, either in the patient's mouth (saliva is an acceptable transport medium) or in a cup of milk which is also an excellent transport medium.[2]

Following replantation, the tooth should be stabilized for at least 2 weeks during which the endodontic treatment can be initiated (ie, 10–14 days). The only exception to including root canal treatment in the management of an avulsed tooth is if it is an immature tooth with a wide open apex, in which revascularization is desirable and may occur. Close monitoring is essential, because infection-related inflammatory root resorption can be very aggressive if it takes place, particularly in young teeth.

EMERGENCY PROCEDURES AND KITS

For the type of dental injuries described above, emergency treatment falls into three categories: Splinting, reattachment of crown fragments, and vital pulp therapy to protect the pulp. Described here will be the procedures and the materials used; mate-rials that can be assembled as kits for use when the need arises.

Splinting of Traumatized Teeth

It is now recognized that one type of splint can be used for all dental injuries requiring stabilization.[3] The type of splint indicated is a nonrigid, flexible splint that permits

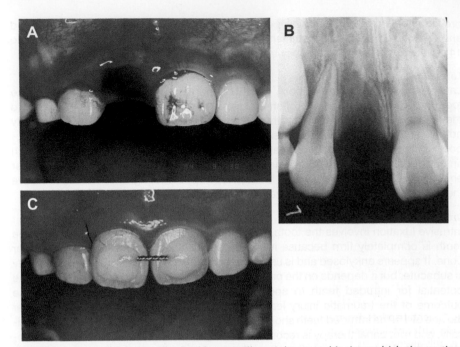

Fig. 6. (*A*) A young patient has avulsed her maxillary right central incisor, which the mother took to the dentist. (*B*) The radiograph reveals no alveolar fracture or tooth fragments left in the socket. (*C*) The tooth has been replanted and splinted. Note that the gingival tissues have been sutured for better adaptation around the tooth. (*Courtesy of* M. Tsukiboshi, DDS, Amagun, Japan.)

physiologic movement of the healing teeth (**Fig. 7**). Alveolar fractures, however, are not included and are currently stabilized with a rigid fixation. The purpose for using a nonrigid splint is to reduce the risk of resorption.[1,4] Including all dental injuries requiring stabilization in one type of splinting protocol simplifies the management of traumatic injuries.

The only variation in the use of the dental splint is in the length of time of stabilization. **Table 1** shows the recommended time periods for the various types of injuries; however, variations may apply and the dentist's clinical judgment must prevail in the various case scenarios.

There are several techniques for applying a splint to the crowns of teeth. Two common techniques are (1) splints made with unfilled resin, and (2) splints made by bonding of a thin orthodontic wire across the crowns of the teeth to be included in the splint.

The flexible resin splint is constructed by etching a small spot on the teeth to be included in the splint, on the labial surfaces of maxillary anterior teeth and lingual surfaces of mandibular anterior teeth. The description assumes anterior teeth because they are involved most often in dental trauma; the techniques described can also be applied to posterior teeth, if indicated. Care should be taken to avoid etching interproximally, because it will result in difficulty in splint removal. The number of teeth to be included in the splint should be the injured tooth/teeth and at least one tooth on either side. After the etching, a bonding agent is applied to the small etched spots, followed by application of an unfilled resin that is subsequently cured. The unfilled resin does not become rigid and brittle when it cures, but retains a slight flexibility which allows physiologic mobility for the teeth.

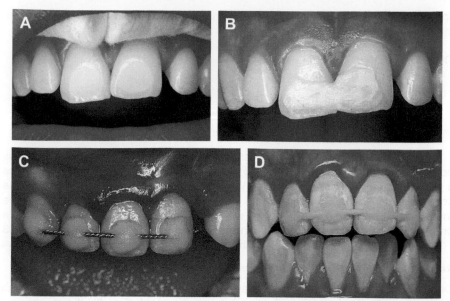

Fig. 7. Dental splints for traumatic dental injuries. (*A*) In preparation for placing a splint made with unfilled resin, the labial surfaces of the central incisors have been acid etched. It is only necessary to etch a small area on the labial surface, making removal easier. (*B*) The unfilled resin has been placed on the labial surfaces and cured. (*C*) An example of a wire splint. For optimal flexibility the wire can be quite thin. (*D*) The use of a nylon line (eg, a fishing line) has been popular, but a thin orthodontic wire is usually easier to manage. (Fig. 7C, D *courtesy of* S. Curiel, DDS, Leon, Mexico.)

Flexible resin splint[1]
- Light cure unit
- Unfilled resin (temporary crown material)
- Acid-etch agent
- Bonding agent

The thin wire splint also allows some minimal movement of the teeth. Similarly to the flexible resin splint, small spots are etched on the labial or lingual surfaces of the teeth to be included in the splint. After placing a small amount of resin, filled or unfilled, to one of the nontraumatized teeth, the wire can be embedded in the resin, which is then cured. The same step is followed for attaching the wire to all the teeth to be

Table 1 Length of time for stabilization	
Subluxation	2 weeks
Extrusive luxation	2 weeks
Avulsion	2 weeks
Lateral luxation	4 weeks
Root fracture (middle third)	4 weeks
Root fracture (cervical third)	Up to 4 months

Data from Flores MT, et al. Guidelines for the management of traumatic dental injuries. International Association of Dental Traumatology. Available at: http://www.iadt-dentaltrauma.org. 2007. Accessed June 15, 2009.

splinted. The small diameter of the orthodontic wire to be used allows for a minimal amount of tooth mobility.

Thin wire splinting[3]
- Light cure unit
- Restorative composite
- Acid-etch agent
- Bonding agent
- Flexible stainless steel ortho-wire, .03 or .04 mm

The splint can be easily removed when indicated, and the spot where the resin was bonded to the tooth can be polished. To remove the splint, if a wire was used, first use a pin or ligature cutter to cut the wire. With a straight diamond bur (eg, # 7901), the composite can be removed from the enamel surface. Next, the enamel surface must be polished. This can be done with a disposable prophy cup and medium prophylactic paste. The final polish can be done with a polishing high speed # 383 FG bur. The goal is to leave a tooth with a smooth and clean enamel surface.

Reattachment of Fractured Crown Fragments

One of the numerous benefits of the development of dental bonding techniques has been the ability to reattach a fractured crown fragment (**Fig. 8**). It has become a successful dental procedure that provides an excellent option for treating complicated and uncomplicated crown fractures.[1,5–9]

Reattaching a fractured tooth fragment is a procedure that can be done in a short period of time. The fractured segment should ideally have been kept moist for the best result; if the patient brings it dry, it can be place in water until it is ready to be attached. The remaining tooth crown and the broken fragment must be cleaned to

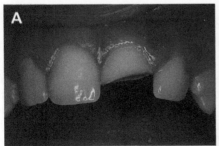
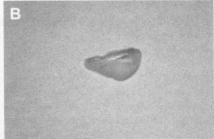
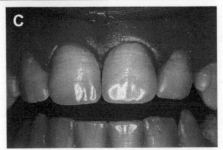

Fig. 8. (*A*) Crown fracture in which the broken fragment (*B*) was saved. Reattachment of the broken fragment can be done with dentin bonding agents, producing a very esthetic and functional result (*C*). (*Courtesy of* Anthony DiAngelis, DDS, Minneapolis, Minnesota.)

remove any debris from the traumatic accident. While local anesthetic is not necessary, it may be more comfortable for the patient.

Materials for reattachment[10]
- Acid-etch agent
- Bonding agent
- Flowable composite
- Light cure unit
- # 7901 high speed bur
- Medium prophy paste
- # 383 FG high speed polishing bur

After drying the tooth and the crown fragment gently with air syringe, the etching gel can be placed on both for 30 seconds, after which it is rinsed off with water and air dried. Next, the bonding agent is applied to the tooth and the fragment and dried with smooth air spray for 5 seconds and then cured with a curing light. Flowable composite resin can then be placed on the tooth and the broken fragment and fitted together like a sandwich.[10] Using the curing light, the composite is cured followed by polishing with a # 7901 high speed bur, and then with medium prophy paste. After that, a #383FG high speed bur can be used to produce a high polish.

Vital Pulp Therapy

Complicated crown and crown-root fractures require attention to the exposed pulp. In adults with fully formed teeth, one would expect that in most cases root canal treatment will be included in the total treatment plan. It is, however, very possible to treat a mature tooth in a manner similar to that recommended for immature, developing teeth. In particular, if the mature tooth is going to be restored by reattaching the broken fragment or by building up the crown using composite resin, it is not unreasonable to preserve the vitality of the pulp. If, however, a prosthetic crown is recommended, it may be prudent to extirpate the pulp and fill the canal to avoid the risk of having to perform root canal treatment through a porcelain crown. Young, developing teeth should be given the benefit of vital pulp therapy. The technique is described elsewhere in this issue.

SUMMARY

The old boy scout motto, "always prepared," can be beneficially applied to the management of dental trauma. A large number of dental injuries occur every year, primarily in the 7- to 15- year age group.[1,11,12] Preserving the natural dentition during that time period is critically important, because tooth loss at an early age presents significant lifelong dental problems.

Being prepared to manage an emergency can make the difference between tooth loss and a successful outcome. Two factors contribute to achieving the better outcome: knowledge of the essentials of dental traumatology, and being prepared with the dental materials needed for appropriate treatment. It is the hope of the authors that these factors are clearly elucidated in this article.

REFERENCES

1. Andreasen JO, Bakland LK, Andreasen FM, et al. Traumatic dental injuries. A manual. 2nd edition. Oxford: Blackwell Munksgaard; 2003. p. 8–9, 16, 17, 26–7, 48–9, 56–7.

2. Blomlöf L, Otteskog P. Viability of human periodontal ligament cells after storage in milk or saliva. Scand J Dent Res 1980;88:436–40.
3. Oikarinen K. Tooth splinting: a review of the literature and consideration of the versatility of a wire-composite splint. Endod Dent Traumatol 1990;6:237–50.
4. Gigon S, Peron JM. Semi-rigid bracket splinting of teeth after traumatic luxation. Rev Stomatol Chir Maxillofac 2000;5:272–5.
5. Andreasen JO, Andreasen FM, editors. Textbook and color atlas of traumatic injuries to the teeth. 3rd edition. Copenhagen: Munksgaard; 1993. p. 517–85.
6. Yilmaz Y, Zehir C, Eyuboglu O, et al. Evaluation of success in the reattachment of coronal fractures. Dent Traumatol 2008;24:151–8.
7. Demarco FF, de Moura FRR, Tarquinio SBC, et al. Reattachment using a fragment from an extracted tooth to treat complicated coronal fracture. Dent Traumatol 2008;24:257–61.
8. Simonsen RJ. Restoration of a fractured central incisor using original tooth fragment. J Am Dent Assoc 1982;105:646–8.
9. DiAngelis AJ, Jungbluth M. Reattaching fractured tooth segments: an esthetic alternative. J Am Dent Assoc 1992;123:58–63.
10. Magne P, Belser U. Bonded porcelain restoration in the anterior dentition. A biomimetic approach. Hanover Park (IL): Quintessence Publishing; 2003. p. 118–9.
11. Andreasen JO, Bakland LK, Andreasen FM, et al. Traumatic intrusion of permanent teeth. Part 1. An epidemiological study of 216 intruded permanent teeth. Dent Traumatol 2006;22:90–8.
12. Andreasen JO, Bakland LK, Matras RC, et al. Traumatic intrusion of permanent teeth. Part 2. A clinical study of the effect of pre-injury and injury factors, such as sex, age, stage of root development, tooth location, and extent of injury including number of intruded teeth on 140 intruded permanent teeth. Dent Traumatol 2006;22:83–9.

Index

Note: Page numbers of article titles are in **boldface** type.

Dent Clin N Am 53 (2009) 761–766
doi:10.1016/S0011-8532(09)00087-1
0011-8532/09/$ – see front matter © 2009 Elsevier Inc. All rights reserved.

dental.theclinics.com

United States Postal Service

Statement of Ownership, Management, and Circulation
(All Periodicals Publications Except Requester Publications)

1. Publication Title	2. Publication Number	3. Filing Date
Dental Clinics of North America	5 6 6 - 4 8 0	9/15/09

4. Issue Frequency	5. Number of Issues Published Annually	6. Annual Subscription Price
Jan, Apr, Jul, Oct	4	$207.00

7. Complete Mailing Address of Known Office of Publication (Not printer) (Street, city, county, state, and ZIP+4®)

Elsevier Inc.
360 Park Avenue South,
New York, NY 10010-1710

Contact Person

Stephen Bushing

Telephone (Include area code)

215-239-3688

8. Complete Mailing Address of Headquarters or General Business Office of Publisher (Not printer)

Elsevier Inc., 360 Park Avenue South, New York, NY 10010-1710

9. Full Names and Complete Mailing Addresses of Publisher, Editor, and Managing Editor (Do not leave blank)

Publisher (Name and complete mailing address)

John Schrefer, Elsevier, Inc., 1600 John F. Kennedy Blvd. Suite 1800, Philadelphia, PA 19103-2899

Editor (Name and complete mailing address)

John Vassallo, Elsevier, Inc., 1600 John F. Kennedy Blvd. Suite 1800, Philadelphia, PA 19103-2899

Managing Editor (Name and complete mailing address)

Catherine Bewick, Elsevier, Inc., 1600 John F. Kennedy Blvd. Suite 1800, Philadelphia, PA 19103-2899

10. Owner (Do not leave blank. If the publication is owned by a corporation, give the name and address of the corporation immediately followed by the names and addresses of all stockholders owning or holding 1 percent or more of the total amount of stock. If not owned by a corporation, give the names and addresses of the individual owners. If owned by a partnership or other unincorporated firm, give its name and address as well as those of each individual owner. If the publication is published by a nonprofit organization, give its name and address.)

Full Name	Complete Mailing Address
Wholly owned subsidiary of	4520 East-West Highway
Reed/Elsevier, US holdings	Bethesda, MD 20814

11. Known Bondholders, Mortgagees, and Other Security Holders Owning or Holding 1 Percent or More of Total Amount of Bonds, Mortgages, or Other Securities. If none, check box ☐ None

Full Name	Complete Mailing Address
N/A	

12. Tax Status (For completion by nonprofit organizations authorized to mail at nonprofit rates) (Check one)
The purpose, function, and nonprofit status of this organization and the exempt status for federal income tax purposes:
☐ Has Not Changed During Preceding 12 Months
☐ Has Changed During Preceding 12 Months (Publisher must submit explanation of change with this statement)

PS Form 3526, September 2007 (Page 1 of 3 (Instructions Page 3)) PSN 7530-01-000-9931 PRIVACY NOTICE: See our Privacy policy in www.usps.com

---

13. Publication Title	14. Issue Date for Circulation Data Below
Dental Clinics of North America	July 2009

15. Extent and Nature of Circulation			Average No. Copies Each Issue During Preceding 12 Months	No. Copies of Single Issue Published Nearest to Filing Date
a. Total Number of Copies (Net press run)			1908	1827
b. Paid Circulation (By Mail and Outside the Mail)	(1)	Mailed Outside-County Paid Subscriptions Stated on PS Form 3541. (Include paid distribution above nominal rate, advertiser's proof copies, and exchange copies)	864	811
	(2)	Mailed In-County Paid Subscriptions Stated on PS Form 3541 (Include paid distribution above nominal rate, advertiser's proof copies, and exchange copies)		
	(3)	Paid Distribution Outside the Mails Including Sales Through Dealers and Carriers, Street Vendors, Counter Sales, and Other Paid Distribution Outside USPS®	390	393
	(4)	Paid Distribution by Other Classes Mailed Through the USPS (e.g. First-Class Mail®)		
c. Total Paid Distribution (Sum of 15b (1), (2), (3), and (4))		►	1254	1204
d. Free or Nominal Rate Distribution (By Mail and Outside the Mail)	(1)	Free or Nominal Rate Outside-County Copies Included on PS Form 3541	64	59
	(2)	Free or Nominal Rate In-County Copies Included on PS Form 3541		
	(3)	Free or Nominal Rate Copies Mailed at Other Classes Through the USPS (e.g. First-Class Mail)		
	(4)	Free or Nominal Rate Distribution Outside the Mail (Carriers or other means)		
e. Total Free or Nominal Rate Distribution (Sum of 15d (1), (2), (3) and (4))		►	64	59
f. Total Distribution (Sum of 15c and 15e)		►	1318	1263
g. Copies not Distributed (See instructions to publishers #4 (page #3))		►	590	564
h. Total (Sum of 15f and g)		►	1908	1827
i. Percent Paid (15c divided by 15f times 100)			95.14%	95.33%

16. Publication of Statement of Ownership
☐ If the publication is a general publication, publication of this statement is required. Will be printed in the October 2009 issue of this publication. ☐ Publication not required

17. Signature and Title of Editor, Publisher, Business Manager, or Owner	Date
Stephen R. Bushing	September 15, 2009
Stephen R. Bushing – Subscription Services Coordinator	

I certify that all information furnished on this form is true and complete. I understand that anyone who furnishes false or misleading information on this form or who omits material or information requested on the form may be subject to criminal sanctions (including fines and imprisonment) and/or civil sanctions (including civil penalties).

PS Form 3526, September 2007 (Page 2 of 3)

Moving?

Make sure your subscription moves with you!

To notify us of your new address, find your **Clinics Account Number** (located on your mailing label above your name), and contact customer service at:

Email: journalscustomerservice-usa@elsevier.com

800-654-2452 (subscribers in the U.S. & Canada)
314-447-8871 (subscribers outside of the U.S. & Canada)

Fax number: 314-447-8029

Elsevier Health Sciences Division
Subscription Customer Service
3251 Riverport Lane
Maryland Heights, MO 63043

*To ensure uninterrupted delivery of your subscription, please notify us at least 4 weeks in advance of move.

Printed and bound by CPI Group (UK) Ltd, Croydon, CR0 4YY

03/10/2024

01040463-0013